EAT, DRINK AND BE MERRY!

BY

TUULA E TUORMAA

Basic principles of illness prevention and treatment
using Nutritional and Environmental Medicine

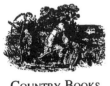

COUNTRY BOOKS

Published by Country Books
Courtyard Cottage, Little Longstone, Bakewell, Derbyshire DE45 1NN England

British Library Cataloguing-in-Publication Data
A CIP catalogue record for this book is available from the British Library

ISBN 1 898941 52 1

All nutritional, medical and health information in this book is based on
research studies and is therefore intended as an information source only.
As each patient is unique, this book is not to be used as a self-treatment
quide but only as a general information source when working with one's
own health practitioner. Neither the author nor the publisher can assume
any medical or legal responsibility for inappropriate use of the information
this book contains.

In memory of my father Eko Tuormaa

DEDICATION

This book is dedicated to the outstandingly perceptive leader of a group of American Indians who inspired these immortal words: "This we know, the earth does not belong to man, man belongs to the earth. Whatever befalls the earth, befalls the sons of earth. Man did not weave the web of life; he is merely a strand in it. Whatever he does to the web, he does to himself." (Chief Seattle 1854)

SELECTED WORKS BY THE SAME AUTHOR

2000   Chromium, Selenium, Copper and Other Trace Minerals in Health and Reproduction. Journal of Orthomolecular Medicine, 15 (3): 145-156 Canada.

1998   The Vitamin B6 Controversy (Memorandum E10) Agriculture Committee, Fifth Report, House of Commons Stationery Office, London, UK.

1996   The Adverse Effects of Alcohol on Reproduction. Journal of Nutritional & Environmental Medicine, 6 (4): 379-391, UK

Adverse Effects of Manganese Deficiency on Reproduction and Health: A Literature Review. Journal of Orthomolecular Medicine, 11 (2): 69-79, Canada.

1995   The Adverse Effects of Tobacco Smoking on Reproduction and Health: A Review from the Literature. Nutrition and Health, 10:105-120, UK.

Adverse Effects of Agrochemicals on Reproduction and Health: A Brief Review from the Literature. (Submission to the Pesticide Safety Directorate and Veterinary Medicines Directorate, March 1995) Journal of Nutritional & Environmental Medicine, 5 (4): 363-366, UK.

Adverse Effects of Zinc Deficiency: A Review from the Literature. Journal of Orthomolecular Medicine, 10 (3/4): 149-164, Canada.

1994.   Adverse Effects of Genito-urinary Infections with Particular Reference to Fertility and Pre-conceptional Care. Journal of Nutritional Medicine, 4 (3): 351-361, UK.

The Adverse Effects of Lead. Journal of Nutritional Medicine, 4 (4): 449-461, UK.

Adverse Effects of Food Additives on Health: With a special emphasis on Childhood Hyperactivity. Journal of Orthomolecular Medicine, 9 (4): 225-246, Canada.

1991   An Alternative to Psychiatry. The Book Guild, Ltd., UK

1988.   A Brief Review of the Immune System and its Function in relation to: Post Viral Fatigue Syndrome (ME), Non-antibody mediated Allergy, Autoimmunity and Immune Deficiency. Nutrition and Health,6 (1): 53-62, UK.

Some studies above can be viewed on the following website:
www.foresight-preconception.org.uk

CONTENTS

ACKNOWLEDGEMENTS

First and foremost, I like to acknowledge the following pioneering researchers and writes on nutritional medicine who are no longer with us; Dr Carl Pfeiffer, Dr Linus Pauling, Sir Robert McCarrison, Professor John Yudkin, Dr Theron Randolph and Dr Richard Mackarness.

I would like to thank especially Dr Abram Hoffer, the editor of the Journal of Orthomolecular Medicine, Professr Derek Bryce-Smith, Department of Chemistry, University of Reading, and Edward Goldmith, the editor of The Ecologist, for having helped me in so many ways during my research projects.

My special gratitude goes to Sir Charles Jessel, The Pelegrin Trust, Edward Goldsmith and Chistopher Gammon for financial support towards the cost of publication of this book. I also like to thank Nim Barnes, Brian Matthews and Jane Gavey for helping me to revise my typescript.

Furthermore, I acknowledge the following doctors, writers and researchers whose work had influence on my research results: Dr Abram Hoffer, Professor Derek Bryce-Smith, Dr Stephen Davies, Nim Barnes, Vicky Colquhoun, Sally Bunday, Dr Vernon Coleman, Lynn Payer, Charles Medawar, Amelia Nathan-Hill, Patrick Holford, Doris Jones, Lynne McTaggart, Martin Budd, Dr Vicky Rippere, Dr Stephen Schoenthaler, Dr Alexandra Schauss, Leon Chaitow, Dr David Horrobin and Dr Merwyn Werbach. There are literally hundreds of others but brevity does not permit me to mention everyone. And last, but not least, I like to thank my dearest friends, particularly Thea, Brian, Jane, Mike, Topper and my Pyry-brother's wonderful music for perking me up when my writing was letting me down.

FOREWORD

Life and its environment are two faces of the same coin; one can not exist without the other, even though the environment came first. There is a continuous interaction, a dance of attraction and repulsion. Life modifies the environment, as it did when it created enough oxygen to force most life to become aerobic, but the changes in the environment also force life to adapt to these changes or to perish. The end point is a stable equilibrium, but this may be short lived or may last for eons of time. Changes can occur very quickly or require millions of years.

Life is driven by special basic needs such as for food, shelter, the need to reproduce, for relationships if the life is human, and for knowledge. In the quest to meet these needs action is taken, but the consequences of this action can usually not be foreseen. The effect of these actions will range from very beneficial to extremely destructive. When our ancestors began the move from trees to the plains, vast new opportunities arose but also vast totally unforseen dangers. Our arboreal ancestors did not know that on the plains they would have much more trouble getting enough vitamin C and that one of the major evils of their move would be world-wide sub-clinical scurvy. It was, and probably still is, impossible to accurately foresee the consequences of such major exploratory moves. But it was our nature to makes these moves. Perhaps there is no other way.

If the toddler knew that learning to walk would be accompanied by many falls and pain, he might decide that it would be better to avoid learning that art. Generally explorers are optimistic when they do their explorations. They ignore potential dangers.

If, in 1904, my father had decided not to move from Europe to the cold, bland plains of Saskatchewan because it would be too dangerous, I probably would not be here. This may be a positive or negative consequence depending upon one's point of view. He foresaw only the potential advantages and played down the dangers of that move. Thus, the innovators, the explorers, the most adventuresome, make changes they are interested in, and their society, if persuaded of the correctness of these activities, will follow. The dangers of that move may become apparent only many years later. They will then be sorry that the moves were made but may have extreme difficulty correcting the situation.

The Japanese Navy, over 100 years ago, fed their sailors polished rice. It was cheaper, more palatable and stored better. They did not know that this would create an epidemic of beri-beri among the sailors. This was the negative product of this move. But there was also a positive product. It led to the discovery of the anti beri-beri vitamin, thiamin, and led to the development of the vitamin as prevention paradigm which reached its zenith about 40 years ago.

And so it has gone on, from one move in our nutrition to another, each followed by negative and positive products of that move. The elimination of coarse fibre and germ from our bread was heralded as a major improvement for mankind, so good that for a long time only the nobility and wealthy could afford to eat it. The negative consequences, the Saccharine Disease, and many accompanying illnesses such as constipation, cancer, diabetes, etc., only came many years later. Every change in our food supply designed to enhance its commercial appeal, was followed many years later by the realization that the end product was the deterioration of our general health. Today at least fifty percent of our population suffer from one or more chronic diseases.

But we have gained a lot of useful information. All the vitamins have been discovered and studied. We know the role of the minerals, the other food components, and we know how to put them together to ensure that our food is nutritious. We know that individuals differ, and that different nutrient needs are present. We know that even though more people live longer, it is often with the heavy burden of senility, both physical and mental.

With all the changes we have made, it is clear that modern societies have been subjected to a massive experiment on the effect on general health of the massive deterioration of food supply, away from the kind of food to which we have adapted in the dance with the environment over millions of years. Over the past 100 years we have departed too far from that dance, and unless we come together again the amount of increase in disease will be exponential. We have cancer, heart disease, arthritis, diabetes, a pandemic of viruses and infectious diseases, but in my opinion we ain't seen nothing yet, unless we reverse the process now underway for so many years, by returning to our bodies the food which will nourish us. Perhaps this is nature's way of reducing the population.

We know what we must do. We must revert back to an interactive system in which the food to which we were adapted is restored but modified in the light of modern knowledge, with improvements that have been shown over many years to be safe such as the addition of iodine to salt, the addition of folic acid to flour, and so on. This book by Ms Tuormaa describes the consequences of having created the maladaptation between our food and our needs, and what we must do to get it restored. Ms Tuormaa's book is well organized, documented with the evidence from medical literature which supports the position she has taken.

Unless we begin the changes that are dicussed, the general health of nations will deteriorate more and more. It will hit nations of peoples coming into the modern current nutrition the hardest, for they will not have had time in which to make even the slightest adaptation. The Inuit in Nothern Canada, the Third World, and nations that are beginning to emulate the worst nutrition habits of our industrialized countries; these are some of the people on earth who will in the next twenty years pay the price we have been paying for the past forty years. This is a warning.

Abram Hoffer MD PhD FRCP (C)

10

INTRODUCTION

My reason for becoming interested in nutritional and environmental medicine stems from my own medical history. It began in the early 1960s when I first started to suffer from repeated bouts of half-fainting sensations which involved palpitations, blurred vision, shaking and difficulties with co-ordination. When I finally decided to see a doctor he diagnosed me as suffering from anxiety neurosis for which I was prescribed tranquillising medication. The next few years were spent travelling all over the world. In all the countries where I lived for some time, I visited a doctor in the hope that someone could find a cure for my pesistent feeling of ill health.

Unfortunately I did not have much luck on that front. All that happened was that my diagnoses changed from one country to another. In Bermuda I was told that my fainting feelings were caused by cerebral arteriosclerosis, in Canada by anxiety disorder, in Switzerland by low blood pressure, In Beirut by a mild form of epilepsy, in Cyprus by psychosomatic disorder, in Sweden by personality disorder and in Finland by hyperventilation syndrome. Not only did the diagnoses differ from one country to another, so did the treatments, ranging from all manner of pills and potions to breathing re- training excercises. Needless to add that the more diagnoses and treatments I was given, the more baffled I became as to why the same individual, suffering from the same group of symptoms, should receive so many different medical opinions?

11

By the time I returned to England in the early 1980s, I was not only fedup with feeling ill most of the time but also determined to find out what is going on? Having experienced differing opinions from doctors whilst overseas, I was now curious as to whether the same would apply if I were to consult different doctors in the same country. To put this to the test I arranged to see three consultants in London one after another. The first diagnosed me as suffering from anxiety neurosis, the second decided that my ill health was due to Post Viral Fatigue Syndrome (PVFS) and the third informed me that the only reason why I felt faint was because I was suffering from reactive hypoglycaemia (low blood sugar).

As before, all doctors suggested different treatments. I left my first appointment clutching a prescription for tranquillising medication, the second advised plenty of rest and the third explained that the only way to overcome my feeling of weakness was to modify my diet in such a way that my blood sugar remains stable. He told me to start the day with a good protein-based breakfast and to consume a protein-based snack immediately when I felt faint. In addition, he told me not to consume any foods or drinks that contain sucrose (refined sugar). He also advised me to eat little and often to prevent my blood sugar from falling too low. I did what the doctor ordered and have been perfectly well since.

My interest in nutrititional medicine began at this point. I qualified as a nutrition consultant in 1984. However, to be able to practise, I needed both premises and time, but I had neither. All I wanted to do was to continue my studies. Besides nutritional biochemistry, I began to read everything I could find regarding environmental medicine (clinical ecology) which is an integral part of nutritional medicine. As the name implies, environmental medicine concentrates on all toxic factors, whether environmental or drug-induced, that harm our health.

It is impossible to describe the feeling of elation on realising that most illnesses, whether mental or physical, can be prevented, and even treated, by using nothing else but wholesome foods. At long last I also received a satisfactory explanation to a question I had put to my suprised mother when I was about seven years old. Strangely enough

I still remember that incident. What happened all those years ago was that I overheard my mother discussing with friends the wonders of modern medicine and how grateful we ought to be because without medications the human race would soon perish. Whilst this palaver continued I became more and more puzzled. After some serious contemplation, this insolent creature piped up: "Can you tell me please how people managed to live before these medicines were invented?" The silence seemed to last forever whilst everybody's eyes were piercing at me. The awkward situation was finally terminated by my mother's tight voice: "Tuula, I have told you many times not to get involved with subjects you don't know anything about. Please go to your room and behave yourself!" This happened over fifty years ago. I wonder who will be telling me off this time?

To make more sense out of both clinical ecology and nutritional biochemistry, I began to study toxicology, pharmacology, immunology and neurology. At some stage I also started to write articles on my research findings and the rest is history. I decided to apply only one rule when writing this book: "If you can't find a book you want, write it yourself". When I first became interested in nutritional and environmental medicine I was desperately looking for a book which could give just a brief outline on both. I was equally keen to find some explanation as to why nutritional medicine is preferred to orthodox drug treatments.

Considering that nutritional biochemistry, clinical ecology and behavioural toxicology are highly specialised scientific disciplines, it is obvious that in this short introductory book I am only able to scratch the surface of each. I have included a reference section and a bibliography for those who wish to study these subjects in depth. However, before I begin, I would like to apologise for my style of writing which must be very boring at times. I hope you don't mind? After all, this book is not meant to entertain but only to clarify some principles regarding nutritional and environmental medicine. I also hope you don't mind the fact that I have used the term 'he' throughout the text to indicate both male and female?

CHAPTER 1

WE ARE WHAT WE EAT

The reason why nutrition is the best 'medicine' in the world is because we are made of nutrients. The bodies of all warm-blooded mammals, including humans, consist of not much else than a skeleton supporting a leathery bag containing salty liquid and a complicated mass of cells interlocking with one another. To keep the whole show in good working order, all we have to do is to nourish and water it well, keep it in the correct temperature, give it sufficient daylight, exercise and content-ment. To nourish it, we have to give it a selection of foods that contain proteins, carbohydrates and fats. Once digested, these are broken into amino acids, vitamins, minerals and essential fatty acids. Our body needs a continuous supply of these nutritional elements to renew itself and to manufacture all the vital enzymes, hormones and neurotransmitters which are indispensable for its maintenance and repair.

Proteins:
Our body converts proteins to amino acids of which eight are essential because they must be present in the foods we eat. The others, known as non-essential amino acids, our body can manufacture providing that our diet contains the necessary ingredients. Essential amino acids are found in their complete form only in foods of animal origin. Vegans,

who do not eat animal proteins, obtain their essential amino acids by combining plant foods together. The importance of amino acids for health goes far beyond protein synthesis because they also act as precursors in neurotransmission and enzymatic activity.

Carbohydates:

All complex carbohydrates such as whole fruit, vegetables, grains and pulses contain starches, fibre and sugars. Once digested, the body converts plant sugars into glucose (blood sugar) which is our main energy source.

Vitamins:

Vitamins are organic substances intimately involved in all chemical processes that keep us alive. As our body is unable to manufacture them, they must be present in the foods we eat. They are divided into water- and fat-soluble ones. The water-soluble are: vitamin C (ascorbic acid), vitamin B1 (thiamine), B2 (riboflavin), B3 (niacin), B5 (pantothenic acid), B6 (pyridoxine), folic acid and B12 (cobalamin). Biotin, choline and inositol also belong to this category even though they are not considered as 'true' vitamins as they can be manufactured by a healthy body. All water-soluble vitamins are harmless even when taken in excess because the surplus is disgarded through urine.

The fat-soluble vitamins are: vitamin A (retinol), D (cholecalciferol, ergocalciferol) and E (tocopherol). Vitamin A is found in two forms: retinol which comes from animal sources and beta-carotene which is present in plants and which our body converts to retinol. Because both vitamin A (retinol) and D are stored in the liver, an excess of either can lead to a toxic reaction. The plant-derived vitamin A (beta-carotene) is not toxic. The same with vitamin E because it is stored in fatty tissues. Vitamin F, collectively known as essential fatty acids, also belongs to the fat-soluble vitamin group.

Minerals:

The most important minerals our body needs to remain healthy are:

calcium, magnesium, potassium, sodium, iron, zinc, copper, chromium, manganese and selenium. Our body uses some as 'buiding blocks' but the main function of most is to act as catalysts in enzymatic activity. In this respect their roles range from weak ionic enzymatic cofactors to highly specific substances known as metalloenzymes. Enzymes are vital for life because they are needed both to transform foods into energy and to break down proteins into amino acids which our body uses to renew itself. In fact, without enzymes, we would be dead as a dodo.

Nutrition in a nut-shell:
Because we are all individuals our nutritional needs differ from one person to the next. Reasons include: hereditary factors, age, digestive ability, environmental pollution, stress, pregnancy and so on. Also some may suffer from an underlying 'nutritional dependency state' which puts an extra demand on their nutritional needs. In other words, the foods one person needs to remain healthy may not sustain the health of another. However, the diet that contains all the vital health-promoting nutritional elements needed to stay bright eyed and bushy tailed is a wholefood diet to which nothing has been added and nothing taken away.

Fruit and vegetables:
Whenever possible, it is best to buy organically grown produce because agricultural fertilizers are notorious for depleting minerals from the soil and all growing matter contains only the minerals that are present in the soil they are growing on. Another reason for buying organically grown produce is, unlike the commercially grown variety, they are free of toxic pesticide residues which are harmful for health. To preserve their vitamin content, the best method to cook vegetables is to use a steamer. Without a steamer, vegetables should be cooked quickly in a small amount of water which can then be used in soups, stocks or gravies. Potatoes are most nutritious when baked or cooked in their skins and fruit when eaten as fresh as possible.

Meat and fish:
Meat is good for our health providing it comes from organically reared animals. It is not only leaner compared to the meat reared on factory farms but is also free of synthetic hormones and antibiotic residues. Meat is best grilled, roasted or stewed with stock and vegetables. Fish, whether fresh or in tins, is also excellent for our health, particularly the oily variety such as tuna, salmon, trout and mackerel, all of which contain plenty of essential fatty acids.

Cereals:
Providing that you are not allergic to wheat, bread and similar products made of organic wholewheat flour are a good source of both vitamins and minerals. Don't be fooled by bread which is made of refined flour with brown colour added to make it look 'healthier'. Also many supermarkets stock bread made of rye flour which is really tasty. Do not forget the goodness of porridge which can be made from oatflakes, oatmeal, millet, pot parley, polenta (corn), rye or brown rice flakes.

Dairy products:
Providing that you are not allergic to dairy products they are good for health. These include milk, cream, yogurt, butter, cheese and eggs. Those with milk allergy can find alternatives such as goat's or soya milk and products made with them.

Oils:
Make sure that your diet contains suffient amounts of unrefined vegetable oils which are an excellent source of essential fatty acids. Always keep the oils in a cool place and out of sunlight to protect them against rancity. For the same reason you should not use unrefined polyunsaturated oils for frying. Olive oil is better or use a mixture of oil and butter or butter alone.

Foods to avoid:
Avoid foods and beverages that contain refined sugar (sucrose). Most

commercial breakfast cereals are high in sucrose. Purchase only 100 per cent wholegrain breakfast cereals or sugar-free muesli. Avoid consuming an excess of caffeine which is not only found in coffee but also in tea and most cola drinks. Good alternatives are decaffeinated coffee and herb teas. If you like your drinks sweet use honey instead of sucrose. Artificial sweeteners are another alternative but use them sparingly because they are also harmful when eaten in excess.

Avoid foods that contain too many additives and those made from refined flour such as white bread, buns, scones and cakes. Similarly avoid foods made from refined grains such as pasta and rice. Instead, buy wholemeal pasta and brown rice. Avoid foods that contain hydrogenated trans-fatty acids such as margarines and/or commercial cooking oils. Most manufactured foods such as pastries, cakes and biscuits are not only high in trans-fatty acids but also in sucrose so leave them alone.

To stay mentally alert, you should start the day by eating a nutritious breakfast. This should contain fresh fruit, wholewheat bread and some good quality protein such as bacon and/or eggs. Nuts, seeds and pulses are other alternatives.

The healthiest diet is a so-called "Mediterranean diet" which usually consists of fish or meat, lightly cooked vegetables, wholewheat bread and/or pasta, a salad, unrefined vegetable oils and fresh fruit.

Life-long dietary habits are obviously not easy to change so it is best not to try to make all changes at once but allow at least a year for alterations. Remember that evolution, not revolution should be the theme. For example, instead of white bread buy an organic loaf. Replace you sugary snack with an apple or banana and you packet of crisps with seeds or nuts. A gradual improvement in health should reinforce your willingness to continue. However, do remember that nutritional medicine cannot be compared to drug treatments. Unlike drugs which 'cure' your symptoms in a matter of minutes, the effect of nutritional medicine takes time because it treats the whole body chemistry. On average, it will take at least three to six months before any benefits are felt. Some may feel even more ill due to withdrawal symptoms which are associated particularly with trying to give up caffeine-based drinks and foods that contain high amounts of sucrose. However, as with most addictions the symptoms should not last longer than a couple of weeks.

The reason why I decided to start this book by explaining first what constitutes a healthy diet is because I want everybody to know before starting to read the next chapters that even though nutritional biochemistry and behaviour toxicology may sound complicated, eating well to stay physically healthy and mentally alert is the simplest thing in the world!

CHAPTER 2
PHYSICAL ILLNESS

It is estimated that 'an average' western citizen eats every year about 800kg of food and drinks at least 800 litres of liquid. Also, that about 75% of western diets consist of manufactured processed foods. What these foods have in common is that they are notoriously low in vitamins, minerals and essential fatty acids. Although a few vitamins and/or minerals may be added to them during processing, the ratio of these essential nutritional elements to calories is still woefully inadequate to meet most of our nutritional needs. Let's look at the evidence.

A 1995 National Diet and Nutritional Survey on 1,700 children, aged between 1.5 and 4.5 years, revealed that 70% ate high amounts of biscuits, white bread, non-diet soft drinks, savoury snacks, chocolates and crisps. More often than not, the main meal of the day was sausages and/or hamburgers with chips. Further dietary estimates revealed that the majority were deficient in most vitamins, including antioxidant vitamins such as vitamin A, E, C, and beta-carotene. The same with minerals, with the exception of sodium, which is plentiful in salty snack-foods. For example, one child in eight was found to be suffering from iron deficiency anaemia and 72% had zinc intake below the recommended Reference Nutrient Intake (RNI). A further 15% had below the recommended Lower Reference Nutrient Intake (LRNI) which means that 15% of these children consumed so little zinc that it was unable to meet any of their nutritional needs (1).

Another dietary survey studied eating habits of 65 inner city school-children aged 12-13. The study found that most children ate nothing at all before leaving for school. In order of priority, the most consumed foods were: chips, white bread, confectionery, biscuits, cakes, buns and fizzy drinks. The majority obtained their calories from sucrose (refined sugar) and from hydrogenated trans-fatty acids found in most manufactured food products such as cakes, biscuits, pies, etc. Further nutritional analysis showed that the intake of most vitamins and minerals by the majority was below the RNI. Of these, 25% had the intake of the following nutrients below the LRNI: vitamin A, E, B2 (riboflavin), folic acid, beta-carotene, calcium, magnesium, iron and zinc. This means, again, that 25% of these childrens' intake of these essential nutrients was so low that it was quite unable to meet any of their nutritional needs (2).

Yet another survey, conducted by the Health Education Authority on 18,002 schoolchildren aged between 11-16, revealed that the majority had no breakfast before leaving for school. Of the ones who claimed to eat breakfast, cereals and toast were the most frequent choice. Once at school, chips, crisps and confectionery were the most popular food items - some claimed eating up to eight packets of crisps and/or sweet items per day. The intake of sugary fizzy drinks was high, many drinking as many as four or five cans every day. Further nutritional analysis showed that the majority were deficient in most vitamins and minerals. The intake of the following nutrients was found to be especially low: vitamin A, B2, B6, iron, calcium and zinc (3).

Yet another dietary survey questioned the eating habits of 1,302 schoolchildren aged 11-16 years, and highlighted several areas of concern. Again, most children had no breakfast before leaving for school. Fatty and sugary foods such as crisps, cakes, biscuits, chocolates and sweets were the most popular food items. So were non-diet soft drinks, 22% drinking more than four cans every day (4).

Another survey among 15-25 year olds revealed similar findings. Judging by the high consumption of crisps, confectionery and fizzy drinks, and a comperative lack of proper meals, the majority of these young adults were found to be deficient in most vitamins and minerals (5). Similar results was found among 463 university students aged 18-20, the majority having vitamin A, B2, folic acid and iron intake below the LRNI (6).

Not only are most of our young folk living on diet which is very low in most vitamins and minerals, it is the same with the majority of families. For example, an official dietary survey among British households revealed that the consumption of the following vitamins and minerals failed to reach the RNI: vitamin C, beta carotene, calcium, magnesium, potassium and iron (7). Yet another, conducted among 7000 families, shows the following pattern: the purchase of cakes, pastries and breakfast cereals had increased, whilst the intake of many essential vitamins and minerals, particularly calcium, zinc, magnesium, folic acid, beta carotene, vitamin C and vitamin B12 had fallen considerably (8). Other surveys show that in most households, the intake of iron, zinc, magnesium, potassium, beta carotene, vitamin C and folic acid falls below the RNI (9,10).

One could could go on and on, but there is no point. Anyone can see that an average British diet is, on nutritional point of view, an absolute disaster. Though the above surveys were conducted among the British population, the results seem to be similar in all countries where the consumption of manufactured convenience foods is preferred to cooking from fresh ingredients. This is certainly the case in North America. Also in Europe, particularly in the north.

That is not to say these countries are short of food. Just the opposite. Even though there are plenty of foods available, they contain hardly anything but calories (hence the ever-growing obesity statistics) whilst being practically void of all the vital nutritional elements we need to stay physically healthy and mentally alert.

Due to their long shelf life, these manufactured convenience foods are great money spinners for food manufacturers and supermarkets alike. The reason why these 'foods' store practically forever is because they are so short of any nutritional value that no self-respecting weevil, fungi or mould would bother to go near the dreaded stuff. Considering even our smallest of creatures are aware that these foods cannot sustain life, how an earth can we expect them to keep us in good working order?

They don't, not properly anyhow. For example, an official health survey, conducted among 7,200 British adults, shows that 23% of men and 25% of women reported suffering from at least one of the following health problems: heart disease, angina, high blood pressure and/or diabetes (11). Another survey found that serious childhood diseases have increased during the last decade, by an average of 85%. For example, cancers among 5-14 year olds have increased by 197%, endocrine diseases by 88% and cerebrovascular diseases by 100%. Also perinatal diseases (diseases affecting the newborn) had increased by a massive 332% (12).

Most tend to blame these ever increasing illness statistics on a lack of medication, a shortage of doctors, nurses and/or hospital beds, insufficient medical research or whatever else. This is wrong. The only reason why so many are suffering is because we deny our bodies the appropriate nutrients they need to stay healthy. Let's look first at the importance of antioxidant nutrients.

Antioxidants:
The most important antioxidants are: vitamin A, E, C, beta-carotene, selenium and zinc. Some act directly as antioxidants whilst others form a part of antioxidant enzymes such as superoxide dismutase and glutathione peroxidase. All fresh, non-adulterated whole- foods contain plenty of antioxidants. They also contain substances known as phytochemicals which also have powerful antioxidant properties. Our body needs a constant supply of antioxidants to protect itself against free radical damage.

Free radicals:
Free radicals, formed as a by-product of oxygen, are highly unstable molecules with an uneven electrical charge. Though most of the oxygen we breathe is converted to water, a tiny amount neverthless

enters the body chemistry. By being unstable and in order to become stabilized, these free radicals are constantly looking for free electrons to latch themselves on to. They are particularly keen in pairing with unsaturated fatty acids which form a part of our cell membrane structure. When this takes place, our cell membranes turn 'rancid' which is known as lipid peroxidation. In fact, free radicals can damage our cells in a variety of ways. Besides harming the cellular structure, they also have an ability to damage our genetic code (DNA) in a way that our cells begin to grow more rapidly or to die sooner. When the cell growth becomes too rapid, this is often a sign of cancer. In cases where the cells begin to be destroyed sooner than nature intended, this is a mark of premature ageing and other degenerative conditions. It is not suprising therefore that ever increasing research evidence is linking excessive free radical formation with the development of heart disease, cancer and Alzheimer's disease.

But nature is no fool. Since the utilization of oxygen has a potentially destrucive side to it, it has provided a method of protecting our cells against possible oxidative injury. This is where the antioxidant nutrients come in as they have an ability to bond with free radicals before they have a chance to attack our vulnerable cell structure. It may be worthy to note, however, that not all free radicals are harmful. When they are formed by our immune system, they enhance its function.

The formation of free radicals is initated particularly when we are exposed to toxic substances such as to polluted air, water, food, radiation, cigarette smoking and so on. In short, the more polluted our environment, the more antioxidant nutrients our body needs to protect itself against free radical formation. Considering that our modern world is teeming with toxic substances and, referring to the surveys mentioned before, our diet seems to be practically void of antioxidant nutrients, we are literally allowing our body to poison itself. The first sign of 'poisoning' appears when more free radicals are formed than our body is able to destroy. No wonder that so many of us are feeling a bit out of sorts! The only way to reverse this situation is to increase the intake of antioxidant nutrients which can be achieved by eating plenty of fresh fruit and vegetables and/or by taking additional vitamin and mineral supplements.

Heart disease:

The reasons for developing heart disease are many. Some are considered as 'risk factors' and others as 'risk markers'. The main risk factor is unquestionably an inadequate diet. Whereas the list of risk markers is endless, including obesity, lack of excercise, not having siestas, cold weather, high blood pressure, cigarette smoking, high cholesterol and so on. However, none of these 'risk markers' cause heart disease directly. They only add to the probability of worsening the underlying condition.

Cholesterol:

High cholesterol, for exmaple, has been linked, for years, with the development of coronary heart disease. This assumption is incorrect. Cholesterol is not just some frightful substance which we have to get rid at any cost to protect our hearts. Just the opposite. Our steroid and sex hormones are made of cholesterol. So are our bile salts needed for digestion. Also our cell membranes need cholesterol, where it acts as an essential lubrication material to facilitate neurotransmission.

Considering that cholesterol is vital for our health, it is not suprising that our body manufactures it all the time. It also possesses a clever built-in-feed-back-control-mechanism in that, the more cholesterol we eat the less our body manufactures. Likewise, if we do not eat sufficient amounts, it increases its synthesis immediately. The end results is that, in healthy people, body cholesterol remains more or less the same whether they prefer to eat it or allow their body to manufacture it. However, some individuals have unfortunately inherited a defect in this cholesterol controlling mechanism, kown as familial hyper-cholesterolaemia (FH). Anyone suffering from this condition must obviously avoid eating cholesterol-rich foods. Whereas for others, moderate amounts will do no harm.

Cholesterol is a lipid, which is a biochemical term describing all fatty substances. It is carried in the bloodstream as lipoproteins which, as the name already implies, are fats that are combined with protein fractions. Lipoproteins are further divided into sub-groups depending on their density, particle size and composition. The of the most important lipoproteins, at least as far our cholesterol transport is concerned, are high-density lipoproteins (HDL) and low-density lipoproteins (LDL). By being the main cholesterol carriers, they are also known as the HDL- cholesterol and the LDL-cholesterol.

The HDL-cholesterol is often described as 'good cholesterol' because it acts like a vacuum cleaner, picking up any stray bits of cholesterol floating in our blood stream and transporting them dutifully into the liver for further use. The LDL-cholesterol, on the other hand, is termed as 'bad cholesterol' because it is the type that becomes easily 'rancid' or oxidised. When this takes place, the body 'sees' these oxidised LDL-particles as something undesirable and foreign. In order to get rid of the 'invaders', our immune system transforms the oxidised LDL- particles into foam cells which have a gluey surface and therefore have an ability to stick readily on our arterial walls. In short, the more LDL-cholesterol becomes oxidised, the narrower our arteries become. This where, yet again, antioxidant nutrients come in, as they are able to prevent the oxidation of the LDL-cholesterol which is associated with the development of heart disease, clot formation and strokes.

Even though the oxidised LDL-cholesterol can do us harm, in its non-oxidised form it is vital for our health because it is responsible for transporting essential fats around our body chemistry. Also with phospholipids, it forms the two principal lipid constituents needed for our cells to work effectively. In fact, studies have found that LDL-cholesterol governs our cell membranes' viscosity whilst the phospholipid fraction governs their fluidity. Studies have also found that the more viscous our cell membranes are, the more effectively they are able to perform all vital cell-to-cell transport processes including neurotransmission.

Considering that the LDL-cholesterol is intimately involved with neurotransmission, it is not suprising that an ever increasing research evidence is connecting low cholesterol with all kinds of mental health problems including violence, aggression, suicides and even schizophrenia (13,14).

Though low cholesterol has been associated with so many mental health problems, it is suprising that the medical profession is still so keen on prescribing cholesterol- lowering drugs. The best answer for this vexed dilemma can be found in a study which examined several research papers concerning cholesterol lowering trials (15). The study points out that the main reason why the medical profession still considers cholesterol to be one of the main causes for the development of heart disease is because the majority of papers published in medical journals have used as references only supportive evidence, whilst ignoring all the studies that show the dangers associated with low cholesterol. The authors conclude: "Lowering serum cholesterol does not reduce mortality nor is it even likely to prevent coronary heart disease. Any claims of the opposite are based on preferential citation only" (15).

Nothing to add except we really should not interfere with nature. By lowering our cholesterol artificially with medication, all we have done is to exhange the remote possibility of developing a heart disease to becoming mentally ill! Admittedly, some studies have shown that a low-cholesterol diet may slightly reduce overall blood cholesterol levels. However, this will have no benefit whatsoever because whilst reducing the 'harmful' LDL- cholesterol, it similarly reduces the intake of the beneficial HDL-cholesterol. Considering that the protective effect of HDL-cholesterol is twice as strong as the artherogenic effect of LDL-cholesterol, we have done our body nothing but a disservice.

Now more good news. We can always raise our beneficial HDL-cholesterol levels by exercising, by stopping cigarette smoking, by losing weight and by drinking moderate amounts of alcohol. Some studies have found that people who take two or three alcoholic drinks a day cut the danger of a heart attack by one sixth whereas others have shown that up to seven units a day, equivalent to 3 1/2 pints of beer or a bottle of wine, offer a protection (16). Cheers!

Indeed, there is no question that a moderate alcohol intake is jolly good for our health and well-being. Unfortunately the same cannot be said when boozing in excess. Not only will an excessive alcohol intake cause irreversible brain damage, it also ruins our liver. Furthermore, it is associated with an increased risk of developing heart disease and cancer. Also, even in smallest amounts, alcohol is harmful to an unborn child, but more about this subject later (17).

Though alcohol in moderation carries nothing but good news, unfortunately the same cannot be said about cigarettes. Besides nicotine, which is the addictive substance in tobacco, cigarettes contain thousands of toxic chemicals which initiate free radical formation. They are also known to have carcinogenic (cancer producing), mutagenic (damaging the genetic code) and teratogenic (damaging the unborn foetus) properties. Considering how dangerous cigarettes are for our health, anyone who is unable to give up the smoking habit ought take at least plenty of antioxidant nutrients. Vitamin C is of particular importance because just one cigarette smoked depletes up to 25 mg of vitamin C from the body chemistry. Furthermore, to protect against the deterioration of lung damage seen in most smokers, every smoker ought to take additional essential fatty acid supplements. Most importantly, it is vital to know that cigarette smoking is absolutely detrimental to an unborn child, but more on this subject later (18).

Both cigarette and alcohol addiction have a nasty ring to them, let alone other addictions such as heroin, opium and similar. What is suprising, however, is that caffeine addiction is considered acceptable even though is also a well known drug. Caffeine belongs to a group of chemicals known as methylxanthines, also found in tea, chocolate and most cola drinks. In common with other addictions caffeine can lead to a serious dependency. Side effects of excessive caffeine consumption include nervousness, irritability, a feeling of anxiety, headaches, insomnia, tension, nausea, palpitations and irregular heart beat. Withdrawal symptoms are well documented including the symptoms above experienced in a far more intensive form. In the majority, the toxic effects of caffeine are felt by anyone consuming regularly more than 750mg of caffeine per day. One average a cup of coffee contains about

100mg caffeine, a cup of tea about 75mg and one cola drink about 50mg. Considering that caffeine is a strong psychoactive drug, an overconsumption can also lead to severe anxiety states quite indistinguishable from anxiety neurosis and similar anxiety related disorders (19). Enough of addictions and back to fats.

Saturated and unsaturated fats:
A fat is saturated if all its double bonds are bonded (saturated) with hydrogen ions which makes them solid at a room temperature whereas unsaturated fats (oils) have double bonds free which makes them liquid at a room temperature. The unsaturated oils are divided further into monounsaturated and polyunsaturated oils depending on the number of free double bonds they contain. As the names imply, the monounsaturates have only one free double bond whereas the polyunsaturates have several. Olive oil is particularly high in monounsaturates, whereas most other vegetable oils such as sunflower, corn, grapeseed and safflower oil are high in polyunsaturates.

Essential fatty acids:
All non-adulterated vegetable oils contain substances known as essential fatty acids (EFAs). The reason why these are termed as essential is because, just as with vitamins and minerals, our body cannot manufacture them but they must be present in the foods we eat. Several types of EFAs have been identified. Depending on the number of carbon atoms and double bonds, each has a slighty different chemical structure. However, our body is particularly dependent on two types of EFAs. One belongs to an omega-6 fatty acids series which derives from cis-linoleic acid and the other to an omega-3 fatty acid series which derives from alpha linolenic acid. All pure non-adulterated vegetable oils contain omega-6 fatty acids. Evening primrose oil, borage oil and blackcurrant seed oil are particularly high in this element wereas omega-3 fatty acids are found in fish oils and oily fish.

EFAs have many biochemical functions. Besides forming an integral part of our cellular membranes, almost 20% of dry weight of the human brain is made of essential fats. They also act as a precursor for a group of highly reactive and short lived molecules known as prostaglandins (PGs) which are vital for a broad range of our body's biochemical activities including muscle contraction, nerve transmission, hormonal regulation, respiration, immune response, gastric acid secretion and so on (20).

The trouble is that even though we might be eating a diet high in essential fatty acids, it does not necessarily guarantee that our body is able to convert them into prostaglandins. This is because before this transformation is able to take place, the EFAs must go first through several biochemical steps. The first step is an enzyme known as delta-6-desaturase (D-6-D) which acts as the number one gatekeeper during the conversion process. For the D-6-D enzyme to work effectively, it requires the presence of several vitamins and minerals of which vitamin C, B6, B3, zinc and magnesium have been found to be particularly important. Not only that, but this delicate transformation process can further be hindered by other factors including, ageing, toxic chemicals and by an excessive intake of either saturated and/or hydrogenated trans-fatty acids (20).

In short, it doesn't matter which way one looks at the situation, it is hardly likely that many have the required enzymatic capacity to transform EFAs to prostaglandins. This is where nutritional supplements come in, such as evening primrose oil which is high in gamma linoleic acid (GLA) and fish oils which are high in eicosapentaenoic acid (EPA). Their healing properties are based on the fact that both have 'bypassed' the destructable D-6-D enzyme and can therefore be converted into the prostaglandings without difficulty.

An ever incrasing number of research studies have shown that essential fatty-acids are beneficial for treating all kinds of mental and physical disorders. For example, they can lower the LDL-cholesterol (20-23) whilst rising the HDL- cholesterol (24). They can reduce blood pressure (23,25,26), blood viscosity (27) and prevent the formation of blood clots (28,29). They have an ability to dilate blood vessels, to reduce angina pain and to improve exercise tolerance (30-32). They also have been found to be useful for reducing arthritic pain (33) and for improving the immune system function (34,35).

Furthermore, evening primrose oil, particularly Efamol, has been used with great success in treating premenstrual syndrome (36) and atopic eczema (37). Similarly for alleviating symptoms associated with multiple sclerosis, particularly when taken at the beginning of the disease process (38). In addition, Efamol supplements have been found useful in the treatment of alcoholism (39,40), schizophrenia (41-43) and childhood hyperactivity (44,45).

Trans-fatty acids:
Even though essential fatty acids are vital for our health, our foods also contain fatty acids which are definitely not. These are known as trans-fatty acids which are formed when natural oils are processed to manufacture margarines. To make the oils into something that can be spread instead of poured, they go through a hardening (hydrogenation) process when the unsaturated cis-bonds of the oils are saturated with hydrogen ions to form trans-bonds which makes them solid. The same thing happens when cooking oils are heated, to protect them against rancity, substancial amounts of trans-fatty acids are formed during the process. This means that most processed foods such as biscuits, cakes, pies, chips, crisps and so on, contain large amounts of trans-fatty acids.

Ever increasing research evidence is linking the consumption of trans-fatty acids with a whole host of health problems including the development of breast cancer (46) and heart disease. As an example, one epidemiological survey conducted among 85,000 American nurses, reported that those who consumed the highest amounts of trans-fatty acids had a 50% greater risk of developing heart disease compared to those who eat the lowest amounts. The association remained even after taking into the account other known risk factors that are connected with heart disease such as family history, blood pressure, smoking and so on (47).

Dr Ronald Finn of the Royal Liverpool University Hospital wrote an excellent letter to The Times of the harmful effects of trans-fatty acids on human health. He mentions that deaths from coronary thrombosis were rare before 1900 even though products such as milk and cheese were eaten in large quantities. Heart disease statistics only began to rise in the early part of this century which coincided with the introduction of margarine and other hydrogenated lipids in 1909. "Those of us in environmental medicine have warned that the introduction of artificially manufactured fats must pose a potential hazard, and now unfortunately we have been proven correct. The total saturated-fat intake should be reduced but not replaced by artificial fats, to which the body has not achieved evolutionary tolerance as with natural foods. Environmental medicine has a small voice in the medical establishment compared with various aspects of high- technology academic medicine. Perhaps the sheer size of this human tragedy will lead to a change." (48).

Table sugar (sucrose):
The development of heart disease has further been linked with an excessive sucrose consumption. One of the most prominent researchers in this field was the late Dr John Yudkin, Professor of Nutrition of the Queen Elisabeth College, London. When he placed volunteers on a high sucrose diet, he noticed that about one third had an adverse reaction to it. Not only that their insulin production increased but also their triglycerine and blood cholesterol levels. Not only that but sucrose made their blood platelets 'sticky' which is independently associated with heart disease. All these adverse reactions dissappeared as soon as he placed these volunteers on a sucrose-free diet. His book entitled 'Pure, White and Deadly' summarises the outcome of many years of his research experiments (49).

Nutrients that are known to protect against heart disease: First and foremost, make sure that you eat foods that are high in antioxidant nutrients, particularly vitamin C. Not only that it acts as a powerful antioxidant, ever increasing research evidence has shown that vitamin C has the ability to increase the beneficial HDL-cholesterol whilst reducing the harmful LDL-cholesterol. Furthermore, because vitamin C is essential for the manufacture of collagen, needed to maintain healthy arterial walls, it has an ability to reduce blood pressure whilst protecting arteries against atherosclerotic damage (50-52). Vitamin E, another antioxidant, has been found to be highly effective in preventing blood clot formation and reducing intermittent claudiation as well as angina pain (50,53). In addition, studies have linked high homocysteine (amino acid) levels in the blood with the development of heart disease (50,54). High homocysteine can be lowered simply and effectively by taking folic acid, vitamin B12 and B6 supplements.

High blood pressure (hypertension):

Hypertension is not an 'illness' in its true sense of the word but a condition caused by several underlying factors. First of all, as we get older, our blood pressure rises due to natural reduction of elasticity within the arterial walls. For example, when we reach sixty, our systolic blood pressure (the upper reading) is usually somewhere in the region of our age plus hundred e.g. around 160mmHG. Also, our blood pressure will rise if our arteries have become even slightly narrowed due to fatty deposits because to pump the same volume of blood through a narrower pipe needs obviously more force. This is simply the body's natural compensatory mechanism to keep us alive because every organ in the body needs the same amount of blood regardless of the condition of our arteries.

Our blood pressure also depends on the consistency of the blood itself, hormone levels, fluid volume and on the health of our kidneys. Similarly on the body mass. If we are overweight, our heart has to work harder, consequently raising the blood pressure. Our blood pressure will also rise when we exert ourselves or are are under tension. For example, it is not unusual our blood pressure to rise whilst a doctor is taking our blood pressure measurements, which is a well-known phenomenon known as a 'white coat' hypertension.

Not only do the underlying causes of high blood pressure vary, so do the treatments. Some doctors may suggest lifestyle changes such stress reduction and/or losing weight. Others prefer to take a more aggressive line by prescribing drugs such as diuretics, beta-blockers, calcium antagonists or ACE-inhibitors.

High blood pressure can also be lowered by dietary means. For example minerals, particularly magnesium, calcium and potassium have all found to be effective in lowering blood pressure (50,55). Also omega-3 fatty acids, found in flax and fish oils, can lower blood pressure substantially in people with borderline hypertension (50,56). The same with foods that belong to the onion family, especially garlic. Not only that it lowers blood pressure, it also acts as a powerful antioxidant, dilates blood vessels, reduces blood fats and inhibits blood platelets from clumping together (50,57). Yet another way to lower high blood pressure is to reduce the 'stickiness' of the blood, which can be achieved by avoiding foods and/or drinks high in sucrose (49).

In short, heart disease can be prevented, even reversed, by consuming of foods that contain high amounts of antioxidant nutrients, especially vitamin C and E and by avoiding foods high in sucrose and trans-fatty acids. Considering that the 'average western diet' consists of about 75% of manufactured convenience foods which are not only notoriously high in sucrose and/or trans-fatty acids but also practically void of both antioxidant nutrients and essential fats, it is no wonder that our heart disease statistics are forever rising. The majority of us seem to think that we only have to start worrying about heart disease when we are older. This assumption is incorrect. In fact, studies have detected fatty streaks in aortas already in three year old children (58). Similarly, many young American soldiers on whom autopsies were performed during the Vietnam war, were found to be suffering from an advanced form of coronary artery disease (59). As the majority of today's youngsters practically live on not much else but crisps, chips and sticky buns, it does not come as a suprise that the incidence of heart disease among 15-24 year olds has risen in the last decade by massive 100% (12).

Cancer:

Few few diseases generate as much fear as cancer, largely because there are still no effective treatments. The usual treatments for cancer are radiation (burning), chemotherapy (poisoning) and surgery. Although some cancers do respond to these, particularly those affecting children, the 'war' against cancer has been well and truly lost. Despite billions spent worldwide on 'cancer research', the disease is only on the increase (60). Is there anything we could to reverse this catastrophy? The answer is a definite 'yes'. As with heart disease, most cancers can be prevented, even reversed at an early stage, by eating a nutritious diet. To understand this concept it is important to know what cancer is and how it develops.

Cancers represent a collection of abnormalities which have in common a failure to control the normal process of cell division resulting in the cells beginning to proliferate in an uncontrolled way. The development of cancers go through the following stages: initiation, promotion and progression. The factors that initiate cancer are collectively known as carcinogens (cancer producing substances) which have an ability to alter our genetic code (DNA) in a way that our cells lose their ability to renew themselves as nature intended so that they begin to divide without any specific regulation.

Our modern world is literally saturated with carcinogens. These include air pollution from traffic or industrial sources as well as a low-level of electromagnetic radiation from mobile telephones, power-lines, computers, TV sets, microwaves or similar. Also some food additives have been found to have carcinogenic properties. The same with some pesticide residues found in our food and drinking water supplies. The list is endless. In fact, it has been estimated that up to 80% of cancers are caused by being exposed to environmental carcinogens (61).

Considering that nobody in the Western world can avoid by being exposed to these harmful substances, one might wonder as to why some develop cancer whilst others don't? The answer is that the majority do develop tiny pockets of disobeying cell growths every now and then which are soon reverted back to normal. The reason why these people do not develop cancer is largely because these individuals possess a highly effective detoxifying mechanism and immune system function which are vital to destroy any 'rogue' cellular tangles before they begin to grow and proliferate.

Whilst 80% of cancers are caused by being exposed to environmental carcinogens (61), another 70% are believed to be related to diet (62). These findings are not suprising because a cancer is not a simple illness but a multifactorial and multi-stage disease process involving a whole array of events. As far as our diet is concerned, it can act either as a cancer promoter or a protector.

Cancer promoters:
For example, a lack of dietary fibre is connected with the development of colon cancer. Some are linking saturated fats with cancer formation (21). Others believe the culprit could be an excessive intake of trans fatty acids, while others associate the development of cancer with a high intake of refined sugars (63). The latter certainly makes sense because sucrose is notorius in lowering the immune system function which acts as the first line of defence against different kinds of 'foreign invaders' including rogue cellular growths (64).

Cancer protectors:
Numerous studies have shown that a high intake of vegetables and fresh fruit offer by far the best protection against the development of cancer (65). This is not suprising because fresh fruit and vegetables, besides containing plenty of antioxidants, also contain other biochemically active substances known as phytochemicals. Several phytochemicals have been identified to date including phenols, ligans, saponins, carotenoids, chlorophyl, plant sterols, phytoestrogens, flavonoids, allium compounds, isothiocynates and indoles (66). Besides being powerful antioxidants, some phytochemicals are also known to prevent carcinogesis by combining with the cancer producing target sites. All cruciferous vegetables such as broccoli, Brussel sprouts, cabbage, cauliflower, cress, horseradish and turnip are known to have this ability (67). The organically grown variety is by far the best. Not only because it has a far higher mineral content compared to the commercially grown produce but also because it contains no pesticide residues, some of which are connected with cancer formation.

Also, all vegetables that contain allium compounds such as onions, garlic, leeks, chives and shallots have a protecive role. Of these, the beneficial effects of garlic have been most widely studied. The health promoting aspect of garlic is based in its mixture of allicin, disulphide, methyl allyl trisuphide plus in other sulphur-containing compounds which give it its pungent odour. Garlic has been found to have antibacterial properties similar to that of penicillin. The difference between the two is, unlike penicillin which attacks the bacterium like a well aimed rifle shot, garlic is a bit of a scatter-shot. It gets there providing you give it some time. Not only is this humble herb brilliant in protecting us against heart disease but also, by being a powerful antioxidant, it has the ability to destroy carginogenic substances before they can attack our vulnerable cell structure.

When doctors diagnose us as having cancer it is usually well in its progressive phase when it is also very difficult to treat. There are few more contentious subjects in medicine than the role of diet in the treatment of cancer, though its role in cancer prevention is already well established. Anyone interested in this controversial subject ought to read Dr Sandra Goodman's brilliant book entitled "Nutrition and Cancer: The State of the Art" which is based on over 5,000 medical and scientific references. The book does not only contain a whole array of information concerning nutrition and cancer, it also explains all known treatments, both orthodox and complimentary (68).

It looks that the more money and time is spent on cancer research, the more complicated the results become. The 'cancer industry' has already detected most cancer initiators and promoters, assuring that a cure is 'just around the corner'. All one has to do is to look at the press headlines: "Science closing in on cancer", "Stopping cancer in its tracks: Drug companies are racing to develop new cancer therapy", "Cancer researchers predict lifesaving advantages in therapy" and so on. This trumpeting continues regardless that more people are dying of cancer than ever before (69). Those who are lucky not to die prematurely from cancer or heart disease, most seem to live spend their lives suffering from some chronic disability or another (11).

There is no question whatsoever that as long we continue ignoring the fundamental fact that there is no other way to remain healthy but to eat foods which nature has provided, our illness statistics will continue to rise. More importantly, it does not matter how many billions we are prepared to pour out to bolster our ailing 'National Sickness Service' it shall remain as insatiable as ever. Our enemies of today are not guns or bombs but the ravages of ill health which we acquire with what we eat. Though we have managed to develop a highly sophisticated technology, our metabolic requirements are still the same as they were thousands of years ago.

Not only is the health of the British population going rapidly down due to an inadequate diet, the same is happening on the American continent. According to Dr Abram Hoffer who is one of the world's leading experts on nutrition and health: "I do not think that any health care system which ignores the profound effects of nutrition on health and disease is going to make any appreciable difference to the general health of the nation. There has been a real increase in the number of people who become sick, despite the ever increasing amount of money spent on making them well. There will be no solution to the problem of chronic illness until we become aware that only by selection of those foods which will nourish us properly, will there ever be a decrease in the growth of the chronic disease industry" (70). The problem with these highly processed non-nutritious foods is that not only do they make us physically ill, but they also affect our mental state. Let's look at the evidence.

CHAPTER 3

MENTAL ILLNESS

It is estimated that between 2-6 million British people are mentally ill at one point in their lives (71). Others have concluded that one adult in seven suffers from some form of mental illness (72). The same with children. An official survey published in 1994 indicates that, during a five year period, the number of children admitted to psychiatric hospitals has risen sharply. For example, admissions of children below ten years of age had gone up by 42% and among 10-14 years by 65% (71). Also that four out of every ten children are likely to be suffering from mental illness before they mature. Some blame these ever increasing child psychiatric problems on growing poverty whereas others on the breakdown of family values (73).

What is suprising that even though most mental health problems are believed to be the result of social events such as the breakdown of family values, poverty, stress, loneliness, or whatever else, the majority of mental illnesses are neverthless 'treated' with psychoactive medications that are designed to alter the brain's biochemistry. Whilst this practice continues, any suggestion that mental illnesses could result from disordered biochemistry is still largely ignored. This discrepancy makes no sense.

Though the modern psychiatric thinking likes us to believe that our body and brain are some sort of separate phenomenon, they are not. Just like our body, our brain consists of a collection of cells which receive their nourishment from the foods we eat. The only difference is that if we deny our body the nourishment it needs, it expresses its displeasure physically, such as with wheezes, pimples, spots, arthritic pains, cancers, heart diseases and so on. Whereas if our brain becomes undernourished, it affects our thinking ability leading to difficulties with memory, perception and behaviour. In other words, a well nourished and non-toxic brain thinks normally, whereas a malnourished and toxic brain thinks abnormally. In order to understand this concept it is necessary to have some idea of what our brain is made of and how it works.

Over half our brain is composed of fatty substances including essential fatty acids, phospholipids and cholesterol. To keep this 'fatty computer' alive, every single minute over one and a half pints of oxygenated nutrient-dense blood must flow through it. Our brain is surrounded by a blood- brain barrier which allows it to exclude, retain or quicken, the transport of any nutritional substances present in our blood supply. Our brain is almost totally dependent on oxygen and glucose (blood sugar) for its normal function. Although the weight of our brain is only about 2% of the total body weight, it neverthless uses up to 30% of all our energy needs.

Besides oxygen and glucose, our brain takes from the same blood supply amino acids to manufacture neurotransmitters which act as its principal chemical messengers. Similarly, it needs a continuous supply of essential fatty acids, vitamins and minerals which it uses primarily as co-factors (helper substances) during the neurotransmitter activity. Over forty different neurotransmitters have been identified of which the most well known are: acetylcholine, dopamine, adrenaline, noradrenaline, serotonin and gamma-aminobutyric acid (74). Almost every drug used in today's psychiatry (and neurology) has been designed either to inhibit, or to increase, the function of one neurotransmitter or another.

Considering that our brain is almost totally dependent on glucose (blood sugar) as its metabolic fuel, it is obviously the very first organ that becomes affected when our glucose reserves plunge. Those individuals who are prone to frequent low blood sugar falls are diagnosed as suffering from reactive hypoglycaemia. This condition was first described in 1924 by Dr Seale Harris who was awarded the Distinguished Service Medal from the American Medical Association for his pioneering work (75).

Reactive hypoglycaemia:

Reactive hypoglycaemia (low blood sugar) is a clinical condition where the fasting blood sugar is almost invariably normal and is not even abnormally depressed by prolonged fasting, but only falls when we are under stress and/or eat an inadequate diet. Diabetes (high blood sugar) is the opposite. Although diametrically opposed, both conditions are closely related as both stem from the fact that the pancreas, whose main function is produce insulin which stabilises the blood sugar levels, is unable to deal with dietary sugars effectively. People suffering from diabetes do not produce enough insulin, or the insulin they produce is defective, resulting in the blood sugar remaining high. Conversely those suffering from reactive hypoglycaemia are producing too much insulin which leads to frequent blood sugar falls.

Symptoms associated with reactive hypoglycaemia include: weakness, dizziness, faintness, trembling, nervousness, irritability, anxiety, poor concentration, feeling of tension, shakiness, mental confusion, slowness of thought, indeciveness, memory lapses, depression, moodiness, temper tantrums, light-headedness, hyperactivity, tremors, joint aches and pains, dry mouth, excessive feeling of hunger and thirst, nausea, sweating and palpitations. Also, in cases where the human brain becomes momentarily very low in glucose, this can result in the normal and rational thinking- brain shutting off completely, leaving the primitive survival-brain in charge when the person begins to exhibit a bizarre behaviour pattern such as uncontrollable temper outbursts and/ or mindless violence.

The main dietary factor for developing reactive hypoglycaemia is excessive sucrose consumption. This happens because if we load our

41

body frequently with sucrose, our pancreas is forced to produce a constant flow of insulin in order to stabilise the resulting high blood sugar levels. When this has continued long enough, the over-worked pancreas becomes eventually so 'trigger happy' that it begins to produce insulin after the slightest of provocations. It is at this point that reactive hypoglycaemia sets in. After years of producing too much insulin, the pancreas may start to malfunction leading eventually to mature-onset diabetes.

In addition, reactive hypoglycaemia has been linked with not eating a nutritious breakfast which has also been proven in laboratory experiments. In one such experiment test individuals were given a breakfast that was high in sucrose. This resulted in an immediate rise in their blood sugar levels, followed soon by a definite blood sugar fall and symptoms associated with it such as weakness, anxiety and irritability. When the same individuals were given a breakfast high in good quality proteins of the same calorific value as the sugary one, this led to a definite sense of well-being that lasted up to six hours (76). If nothing else, this experiment shows that the best 'medicine' for the treatment of weakness, anxiety and irritability is to consume good quality proteins and to avoid foods that are high in sucrose.

Another problem associated with reactive hypoglycaemia is that each time our blood sugar reserves plummet, our adrenal glands begin to secrete adrenaline in order to release stored glucose (glycogen) from the liver. As adrenaline is the principle hormone that initiates the so-called 'fight or flight' response, it is no wonder that a sudden release of this hormone makes us feel anxious, even to experience mild panic attacks. Furthermore, when our adrenal glands become over-stressed due to a constant demand to produce adrenaline, this can eventually lead to a mild form of adrenal insufficiency which is associated with a feeling of lethargy, weakness, mild depression and low blood pressure (77).

Also all stimulants that are high in caffeine such as coffee, strong tea and cola drinks have an ability to instruct our adrenals to release adrenaline which then nudges our liver to release glycogen from its stores. Nicotine has the same effect. As both have an ability to raise our blood sugar levels this is why caffeine-based drinks and/or cigarettes stop us feeling hungry.

Reactive hypoglycaemia is diagnosed through symptoms and by taking a careful dietary history. The condition can be confirmed in the laboratory using a 5-hour glucose tolerance test (GTT). The main trouble with the test is because it is conducted in such artificial circumstances, the results may not be accurate. However, anybody who suspects suffering from reactive hypoglycaemia can check this at home. There are many self-help books on the subject. The books that I found most useful are Martin Budd's "Low Blood Sugar (Hypoglycaemia) - The 20th Century Epidemic?" (78) and Paavo Airola's "Hypoglycaemia: A Better Approach" (79). Furthermore, Dr Lesser's book: "Nutrition & Vitamin Therapy: The Dietary Treatment of Mental and Emotional Ill-Health" is excellent because it does not only explain how to recognise reactive hypoglycaemia but also other nutritional deficiencies known to lead to mental health problems (77).

Only briefly. The simplest way to self-detect an underlying reactive hypoglycaemia is to alter one's diet for a couple of weeks to see whether symptoms disappear. First of all, start the day with a nutritious protein-based breakfast. Avoid all foods and drinks that are high in sucrose including alcohol. At least, never consume them on an empty stomach but always first eat some good quality proteins. The same with stimulants such as caffeine and cigarettes. It is best to eat little and often as this will assure a regular bood sugar supply. If you start feeling perkier on this diet, reactive hypoglycaemia is a strong suspect. In fact, it has been estimated that as many as one person in four in the Western world is likely to be suffering from the condition (78,79).

It is unfortunate that the majority of the orthodox medical profession is adamant that reactive hypoglycaemia is rare though the evidence points to the contrary. For example, a Joint Report of The Royal College of Physicians and the British Nutritional Foundation on food intolerance and allergies mentions it only in passing (80). It points out that reactive hypoglycaemia is associated with a wide variety of symptoms including hunger, sweating, palpitations, headache, abdominal pain, vague feelings of ill-health and even with bizarre and aggressive behaviour. However, according to the report, claims that low blood sugar is responsible for ill-health in adults have not been substantiated. Similarly, that it is rare amongst children, adding that "despite this, many writers in the lay press have continued to assert that reactive hypoglycaemia is important, particularly in children, because they eat so-called 'junk food'" (80).

One just can't help wondering on what basis the medical profession concludes that reactive hypoglycaemia is a rare and therefore should not be taken seriously? Let's face it, as long they prefer to believe that the condition is largely an invention of the 'lay press' and not much to do with them, it is not suprising that they fail to recognise it in their clinical practice. However, the doctors who have been looking and testing for it, seem to find it often enough, particularly among the criminal fraternity. For example, when Professor Martti Virkkunen, from Helsinki University, Finland, conducted 5-hour glucose tolerance tests and insulin measurements among violent offenders, he found that the majority were suffering from reactive hypoglycaemia (81-83). In fact, ever increasing research evidence is linking reactive hypoglycae-mia as one of the main reasons for impulsive, violent, antisocial and explosive behaviour pattern which can only be corrected by treating the underlying hypoglycaemic tendency (84).

Considering that the human brain is more sensitive to blood sugar changes than other parts of the body, it does not come as a suprise that it seems to be more sensitive to other nutritional deficiencies (84-119). Let's look at the evidence.

Vitamin B1 (thiamine):
When human volunteers were given a thiamine restricted diet, mental symptoms included aggression, irritability, memory failure, loss of concentration, anxiety, depression, apathy, confusion, instability, rest-lessness and unco-operativeness (90). Furthermore, when Longsdale and Shamberger studied 20 youths suffering from sub-clinical thiamine

deficiency, the symptoms included: chronic fatigue, dizziness, blurred vision, sleep disturbances, headaches, nausea, depression, aggression, hostility and poor impulse control. This study points out that the reason why these youngsters were suffering from sub-clinical thiamine deficiency was largely due to their high-sucrose diet which is notorious for depleting thiamine from the body chemistry (91). By the way, the term sub-clinical is used in medicine for any condition where not enough symptoms are present to warrant a specific diagnosis such as in this instance, beri-beri, which is a serious thiamine deficiency disease.

Vitamin B2 (riboflavin):

Unlike thiamine, sub-clinical riboflavin deficiency is rarely associated with mental health problems though this is possible. For example, when volunteers were given a riboflavin-restricted diet, it took about a month before mental symptoms appeared which included: hysteria, hypomania and psychopathic deviation (92). Also, when Carney and colleagues studied 172 newly admitted psychiatric patients, they found that 29% were suffering from sub-clinical riboflavin deficiency (93).

Vitamin B3 (niacin):

The first noticeable signs of sub-clinical niacin deficiency seem to be largely psychological including irritability, emotional instability, loss of memory, apprehension and vague feelings of fear. Maybe one of the best descriptions of sub-clinical niacin deficiency can be found in Dr Green's paper 'Sub-clinical pellagra' which he based on his own observations whilst working near Indian settlements in Canada (94). The majority of his patients with a low-level niacin intake complained of suffering from visual 'zoom effects' where objects seemed to be moving back and forth, becoming smaller and larger, changing shape, leaning over, or becoming distorted. Most felt similar distortions when walking on solid ground. They had an impression that the ground had a sponge-like appearance which was moving forwards, sideways, up-hill and downhill. Many also claimed 'hearing voices'. In fact, the study points out that the symptoms between sub- clinical niacin deficiency and schizophrenia is only a matter of degree as both share the same visual and mental distortions (94).

Dr Green concludes that since niacin has been added to many manufactured food products the obvious vitamin B3 deficiency disease (pellagra) is rarely seen in clinical practice. However, it is quite wrong for the medical profession to assume that once a vitamin has been added to some manufactured foods that this will automatically quarantee that no-one will ever suffer from sub-clinical vitamin deficiency states. In his opinion, this is a strange way to deal with any disease whose very existance depends on nutritional ignorance and, as long as people are unaware of the vital importance of eating nutritious foods, they will only eat what they fancy. Also, 'as long as there are people to whom profit means more than the health of the nation, the poor and the ignorant will be exploited by hucksters peddling puffed wheat, corn-flakes and instant This and That, nearly all at the expense of the protein, vitamin and mineral values of food'. Doctors must have an open mind. As long as they continue in believing that sub-clinical vitamin and/or mineral deficiency states do not exist, they will never be able to diagnose them (94).

Vitamin B6 (pyridoxine):
A sub-clinical vitamin B6 (pyridoxine) deficiency is also associated with psychiatric disorders including anxiety, nervousness, fatigue, poor memory, apathy and depression (95- 97). For example, when Carney and his colleagues tested 64 psychiatric in-patients, most having been diagnosed as suffering from 'affective disorders' which include such diverse conditions as anxiety states, depression, mania and hypomania, they found that 28% were suffering from sub- clinical pyridoxine deficiency (97).

Folic acid and vitamin B12 (cobalamin):
A low intake of either causes anaemia. A severe vitamin B12 deficiency leads to pernicious anaemia which is a rare but very serious clinical condition. Folic acid deficiency causes megaloblastic anaemia

which is characterised by immature and malformed red blood cells. However, before the anaemias develop, both sub-clinical vitamin B12 and folic acid deficiency are associated with a myriad of mental disorders including depression, confusion, mood disturbances, apathy, psychoses, Alzheimer's disease and senile dementia (98-112). Considering that sub-clinical folic acid deficiency appears to be particularly common in those suffering from depression, studies suggest that it is always justifiable, before any other treatment is even considered, to test whether the depression is caused by an underlying folic acid deficiency. Also, because mental symptoms of low vitamin B12 levels can precede, sometimes by years, the actual appearance of pernicious anaemia, it would be prudent if all patients suffering from any psychiatric disorders were first tested for a possible sub-clinical vitamin B12 deficiency. However, considering that pernicious anaemia is an extremely serious condition which can be masked by a high intake of folic acid, it is vital that a correct diagnosis is made first. Whenever in doubt, patients should never be given high doses of folic acid, at least on a long term, without additional vitamin B12 supplements.

Vitamin C (ascorbic acid):
Vitamin C deficiency leads to a serious nutrition deficiency disease known as scurvy. However, before the condition develops, sub-clinical ascorbic acid deficiency is associated with depression, weakness and lethargy (113).

Our mental health is not only dependent on vitamins, minerals are equally important. Take zinc for example, which our body needs for over 100 of its enzyme system functions. The mental signs of sub-clinical of zinc deficiency are known to include: apathy, sullenness, lethargy, depression, irritability, hyperactivity, mood swings, schizoid episodes, anorexia nervosa and senile dementia (114-116). Sub-clinical iron deficiency is associated, particularly in children, with restlessness, hyperactivity, irritability and a reduced intellectual function (117-119). Also other minerals are important but this will suffice. Anyone interested to learn more how inadequate intake of vitamins and minerals can affect our mental state, the best overall guide on the subject, at least in my opinion, is Dr Pfeffer's book "Mental and Elemental Nutrients" (87). Highly recommended!

All we have to do now is to turn back to the beginning of the previous chapter which shows that the great majority of us seem to be short of not only one, but of several vitamins and minerals required for a well-functioning brain. No wonder so many seem to have problems in thinking straight! However, it is our children we really ought to worry about because hardly a day goes by without the media reporting some incident or another connected with our childrens' ever deteriorating behaviour patterns. In fact, the fast deterioration in behaviour among the young is nowadays resembling an epidemic, with symptoms including utter mental derangement coupled with a complete lack of behavioural and self-control. Violence is abhorent in all circumstances, but when teachers are frightened to do their job because of fear of being attacked by pupils it is really the end of civilisation as we know it.

Whilst our teachers are looking for panic buttons, all we seem to be doing is putting the blame for our childrens' ever deteriorating behaviour on all kinds of socio-political influences, such as inadequate parental control, TV and film violence, breakdown of family values, lack of police, 'sin-bins', corrective institutions, an inadequate teaching profession or similar. For example, not that long ago I was watching a television programme where experts were questioned about why our childrens' behaviour is forever deteriorating? And, what best to do to reverse this frightening trend? Some blamed the parents, suggesting that the only way to stop children misbehaving was to demand that parents pay a fine each time their child does something wrong. Some suggested that parents ought to be given lessons in how to bring up their children properly. Others had an opinion that the only way to improve childrens' behaviour was to give teachers the right to inflict physical punishment on the offending child. Others believed that the reason why so many children are unable to behave themselves was due to too much discipline. Some blamed incompetent teachers for lacking the ability to teach, whereas others demanded special schools for disruptive pupils.

This tirade went on for nearly two hours during which nobody mentioned, not even in passing, that one way to help our children to behave is to improve their diet.

Considering that the diet of the majority is lacking most vital nutritional elements needed for a well-functioning brain, the obvious thing to do is to make sure that our children are well fed. As we have seen, most official dietary surveys show that the majority are very short of zinc and iron which can lead to the following mental health problems: apathy, irritability, sullenness, mood swings, restlessness, hyperactivity, disruptive behaviour and a reduced mental performance. Similarly, most surveys show that the majority leave for school without eating any breakfast and, once at school, most seem to be living on not much else but sugary snacks. This being the case, it would not be suprising that most may also be teetering on the brink of reactive hypoglycaemia, symptoms including impulsive, violent and antisocial behaviour patterns. Another problem with foods high in sucrose is that they deplete vitamin B1 (thiamine) from the body chemistry which in turn is known to lead to aggression, irritability, loss of concentration, anxiety, confusion, apathy, instability, restlessness, unco-operativeness, hostility and poor impulse control. No wonder so many children have difficulties in behaving themselves. Most would, if they only could!

A press article, published in 1996 reported that; "More than nine out of ten teachers said they were facing more discipline in the class and one in three said the position was much worse than 15 years ago" (120). I found this particularly interesting because just fifteen years previously the government decided to abolish the then existing official guidelines that school meals ought to provide at least one third of childrens' daily nutritional needs. Soon after, the tuck-shops opened their colourful counters. The food manufacturers are obviously well aware that children are consumers in their own right and so they are also prime targets of advertisements designed to exploit their preferences in food selection. In fact, it is estimated that over half the advertisements during childrens' television are designed to entice our kids to purchase all sorts of non-nutritious edables. Resulting that the tuck- shops are flourishing whilst our children are 'grazing' through the day eating their colourful junk.

It is astonishing why it is that science has come into most aspects of our daily lives but not into problems with behaviour? The science we ought to look at here is nutritional biochemistry. In other words, the only way to help our children to behave is to make sure that the food they eat contains all the nutrients needed for a well- functioning brain. They do not need 'sin-bins' or correction facilities, only a hefty school dinner lady watching over them so that they eat every scrap of wholefoods from their plates!

Some may like to argue that school meals are unnecessary because the responsibility of seeing that children are well nourished belongs to parents. This is unrealistic. After all, in today's economic climate, both parents are usually working and, on returning home, they are often either too tired or otherwise preoccupied to start preparing a wholsesome meal from fresh incredients. In fact, in the majority of households 'grab it from the freezer and bung it in the microwave' is as close as it will ever come to home cooking.

There are also millions of parents who simply cannot afford to feed their children as well as they would like. Many refuse to acknowledge that poverty exists in the developed world, but it does. In fact, it is estimated that as many as two British children in five are living in circumstances described as poverty. Food is not cheap, particularly ready-made meals. It would be far cheaper to cook from fresh ingredients. However, due to declining emphasis on cooking skills in the National Curriculum, many of todays' parents have no idea how to prepare even the simplest of meals from fresh provisions. Considering that today's children will be tomorrow's parents, we simply cannot afford our next generation to remain nutritionally ignorant. The only way to reverse this worrying trend is that, from an early age, all children are taught at school how to prepare basic meals using fresh ingredients. They would not only learn the art of cooking but at the same time they would have loads of fun.

Toxic excesses:

Another science which is linked with mental health problems is behavioural toxicology which concentrates on all the toxic factors that affect the brain's biochemistry. The most well-known behavioural toxin is alcohol (17). Street drugs, such as heroin, morphine and opium also belong in this category. So do heavy metals, such as lead, cadmium, aluminium and mercury (18,121-125). The behavioural effects of lead contamination are perhaps the most widely studied (121-125).

Some of the strongest evidence of how even small amounts of lead pollution can alter childrens' behaviour can be found in a well controlled study conducted by Dr Needleman and his team (125). The results show clearly that the higher the childrens' body lead levels the more disruptive was their behaviour and the less well they were able to perform in all tests concerning learning ability and mental function. The major lead pollution results by being exposed to leaded petrol. Also some drinking water supplies contain high amounts of lead, particularly in houses with old lead piping and where the water is soft and acidic, which literally corrodes layes of lead from the pipes (124).

Also some synthetic food additives are known to act as behavioural toxins, particularly in children (121,126-131). The food manufacturing industry is currently using about 3,800 different food additives of which over 3,600 are used for cosmetic purposes only and the rest as preservatives and processing aids. Considering that a high proportion of the western diet consists of manufactured food products, it is estimated that an average person consumes about 8-10 lbs of food additives per year, some eating considerably more (126).

Childhood hyperactivity:
Obviously most normal children are overactive and inattentive at times but hyperactive children are different. One of the most noticeable differences between a normally overactive child and a child who suffers from hyperactivity is that the former tends to respond to what is said to him whereas the latter seems to live in a whirl-wind world of its own. It is as if he is constantly driven by some mechanised battery which just forces him to go on and on, regardless of the consequences. This

condition is also known by many other names including: hyperkinetic syndrome, Attention Deficit Disorder (ADD), learning disability, developmental imbalance, Attention Deficit Hyperactivity Disorder (ADHD), perceptual handicap and minimal brain dysfunction disorder. As the names already indicate, we are not only dealing with a child who is hyperactive but who also suffers from a variety of learning disabilities (126,127).

The child suffering from this disorder is not only hyperactive but unpredictable, impulsive, destructive, inflexible, uncooperative, defiant, disobedient, aggressive and selfish. Because of his impulsiveness, which the child is unable to control by the way, he may dart over a busy road without taking a blind bit of notice of oncoming traffic. He is also a constant climber of and faller off furniture, trees, balconies, or whatever. In other words, a child suffering from hyperactivity just continues to do the most stupid and extraordinary things which a normal child would think at least twice before even attempting to do.

He also tends to suffer problems with co-ordination resulting in difficulty in tying his shoe laces, buttoning garments, playing ball games, writing, drawing, or doing anything that requires fine motor control (126,127). Furthermore, he is fidgety, restless and lacks any power of concentration whether the task involves eating a meal, playing games or doing school work. Because of his concentration difficulties, his school grades are usually poor though he might have a normal or even a high intelligence. Also, due to his unruly behaviour, he is often written off by teachers as being uneducatable. Considering the wide range of behavioural problems associated with childhood hyperactivity it does not come as a suprise that these children cover the main proportion of all patients seen in child psychiatric practice (126).

The Hyperactive Childrens' Support Group (HACSG) which was formed over 20 years ago, has done a great deal of research on the subject. For example, one of their research projects on 357 hyperactive children show that the majority were already suffering from health problems as infants such as colic, eczema, asthma, catarrh, hayfever, joint pains and frequent ear and/or chest infections. In addition, the majority hated to be fed but demanded drinks most of the time. Also, many shunned motherly contact or affection. Moreover, the study found that most of these hyperactive children had been born to atopic (allergic) families with a history of asthma, eczema and/or hayfever (127).

Food allergy and childhood hyperactivity:

Ever increasing research evidence has shown that an excessive consumption of synthetic food additives and/or underlying food allergies can lead to hyperactive behaviour. Some of the most convincing evidence to that effect can be found in a double-blind, placebo controlled, cross-over trial, conducted by Dr Egger and his team (128). First, they placed 76 severely hyperactive children for four weeks on a so-called oligoantigenic (a few foods) diet which is low in allergenic potential. The diet consists typically of nothing else but lean meat, lighty looked vegetables, fresh fruit and spring water. While on this simple diet, 12 children were completely cured from their hyperactive behaviour and others improved a great deal.

After this trial period was over, the research team wanted to find out which food(s) and/or chemical(s) were responsible for the children becoming hyperactive. In order to do so, all children were gradually re-introduced to their own typical every-day foods when it was found that 79% became hyperactive as soon as they ate or drank anything that contained a food colouring tartrazine (E102) and/or preservatives known as benzoates (E210-E219). Incidently, tartrazine is used widely by sweet and soft drink manufacturers, whereas benzoic acid is found in some jams, fruit-based fillings and fruit drinks.

Even though tartrazine and benzoic acid were the most common substances that provoked hyperactivity, none reacted to them alone. In fact, as many as 48 different foods were found to be responsible. However, the most prominent foods in order of priority were: cow's milk which affected 64% children, chocolate (59%), wheat (49%), orange (45%), hen's eggs (39%) and sucrose (table sugar) (16%).

Now some good news. After the individually offending foods and chemicals were removed from the childrens' diet, not only did their hyperactive behaviour improved but also other symptoms associated with allergies such as headaches and eczema. The study concludes: "This trial indicates that the suggestion that diet may contribute to behaviour disorders in children must be taken seriously..." (128).

A couple of years before the study above, Dr Egger and his team conducted a similar double-blind, placebo controlled food trial among 88 children suffering from frequent migraines (129). The results show that 93% of the children were cured from their migraines after the individually offending foods were removed from their diet. As previously, not only did their migraines improve but also 'associated symptoms' such as abdominal pain, fits, asthma, eczema, recurrent mouth ulcers and hyperactive behaviour. Similarly, as before, most children reacted to several food items. However, the most troublesome substances in order of priority were: cow's milk, hen's eggs, chocolate, orange, wheat, benzoic acid, cheese, tomato and tartrazine (129).

Another important point. The researchers found that even though some children had high serum IgE antibody levels, only three out of the 88 reacted positively to skin prick tests which are used by the medical profession to identify allergies. It was concluded therefore that this type of allergy cannot be diagnosed by conventional allergy tests but only by using a carefully controlled dietary exclusion and challenge which, if not performed under medical supervision, can be dangerous (129).

Food additives and childhood hyperactivity:

Dr Ben Feingold was the first one to introduce to the medical profession the ground-breaking theory that artificial food additives can be responsible for childhood hyperactivity (130,131). Thereafter, the so-called 'Feingold diet' has been used, world-wide, in treating children suffering from this disorder. The diet is simplicity in itself. All one has to do is to remove all foods that contain synthetic food additives from the child's diet and replace them with non-adulterated and nutritious whole-foods. Also, it excludes, albeit briefly, fruits and vegetables that contain natural salicylates such as almonds, apples, apricots, peaches, plums, prunes, oranges, tomatoes, tangerines, cucumber, blackberries, strawberries, raspberries, gooseberries, cherries, currants grapes and raisins. I will say no more about this subject. Anyone interested in finding out how to treat childhood hyperactivity by diet, whether a parent or a member of the medical profession, ought to get in touch with the Hyperactive Childrens' Support Group (HACSG) as they know everything worth knowing about the subject. You will find their address at the end of this book. As a basic guide for parents I recommend a book by Barnes and Colquhoun entitled: "Hyperactive Child, Attention Deficit Hyperactive Disorder: A practical self-help guide to parents" (127).

It is unfortunate that it is always the very youngest who serve as the first casualties of any toxic contamination. The young, newly developing nervous system is particularly vulnerable. Even studies that have been highly critical of Dr Feingold's claims that synthetic food additives can lead to childhood hyperactivity have concluded that the younger the child, the more likely it is that his behaviour deteroriates after eating additive-rich foods (126). Besides acting as a direct toxin, there are other ways that foods high in additives can lead to behavioural disturbances. First of all, most foods high in additives are generally low in most vitamins, minerals and essential fatty acids needed for a well functioning brain. Secondly, many are high in sucrose which can lead to reactive hypoglycaemia and symptoms associated with it.

Food allergy and intolerance:
Though allergies have a hereditary component, this does not necessarily mean that everybody who has inherited an allergic tendency will become allergic. Neither is there a guarantee that those who have no family history of allergy will never become allergic. In fact, ever increasing research evidence is linking the development of allergies to a non-nutrious diet coupled with an excessive exposure to toxic substances. This makes sense. After all, our immune system, which acts as the first line of defence against allergenic substances, needs a con-

tinuous supply of vitamins and minerals to work effectively (132). The same with our detoxifying mechanism which needs a constant supply of antioxidant nutrients to deal with incoming toxins. If we continue to deny our body these vital nutritional elements, not only does our immune system become defective but also our detoxifying mechanism. When this is allowed to continue long enough, our body will eventually become so overburdened that one day it fails to tell the difference between our favourite snack and a wollop of toxic matter. That is when allergies set in. This seems to be the body's way of saying "enough is enough!". As always, it is the very youngest who are most vulnerable because, unlike mature adults, their immune systems, as well as detoxifying mechanisms, are still at an early stage of development.

A medical report entitled "Food Intolerance and Food Adversion", published jointly by the Royal College of Physicians and the British Nutrition Foundation, points out that food intolerance, not allergy, is an appropriate term to use if no immunological mechanism has been identified (80). Also that skin tests, total IgE and IgE antibody measurements are of poor diagnostic value in cases of food intolerance since both can give either false positive or false negative results. It further explains that the only way to diagnose food intolerance is if symptoms disappear with an elimination diet and, if a controlled food challenge leads to a recurrence of symptoms.

The report suggests that the elimination and challenge diet ought to be performed using the following guidelines: A simple diet is given over a period of two, preferably three weeks, eliminating either individually identified foods or, if these cannot be determined, eliminating all foods which are most closely associated with allergic reactions. Whilst the patient is withdrawing from these allergy producing substances, he may experience during the first week uncomfortable withdrawal symptoms which, in some cases, can take up to three weeks. Also, since the adverse effects of certain foods may depend on quantity, the newly introduced foods may need to be taken for two or three successive days before they can be assumed for certainty not to cause an allergic reaction. Furthermore, because delayed reactions to foods

56

are not unusual, new foods should be introduced to the diet only at five or six day intervals. Also, when the patient is challenged with the offending foods and/or chemicals, caution is vital when the tests are carried out on highly sensitive individuals because the reaction can be so severe as to be even life threatening (80). All in all, this section of the report is highly commended for its accuracy.

The report also discussed childhood hyperactivity and clinical features associated with this disorder, including poor concentration, short attention span, impulsive behaviour, resistance to discipline and underachievement at school. However, according to the report, in the experience of most paediatricians, childhood hyperactivity in relation to foods never occurs in isolation but is usually associated with other allergic symptoms such as migraine, diarrhoea, urticaria and eczema. It also refers to the Feingold diet in rather a derogatory manner pointing out that it has been 'extensively encouraged by lay organisations representing the parents of so-called hyperactive children' (80).

In the concluding remarks the report mentions that although food intolerance has gained increasing recognition in recent years, a comparative shortage of adequate scientifically based research evidence, combined with the lack of medical interest in the subject, has resulted in the proliferation of organisations, centres and individuals who offer advice on how to treat food intolerance which has little scientific basis. Also that while doctors have made some advances in recent years in understanding food intolerance, their knowledge of the aetiology, reliable diagnostic methods and satisfactory forms of treatment is still inadequate. What they would particularly like is to define the mechanism, immunological or non-immunological, by which foods are causing a reaction in susceptible individuals. They would further like to know whether maternal diet and/or environmental factors can affect the immune system function in such a way that the person becomes intolerant to foods in later years. Similarly, they would like to determine the similarities and the differences between patients who suffer from food intolerance and of those who have been diagnosed as being mentally ill (80).

During all the years I have been concentrating on my work, I have not come across another study with so many conflicting messages as the one above. Whilst it gives the impression that the medical profession knows precisely how to diagnose food intolerance, it is neverthless not prepared to do anything about it. At least not until they have established whether the condition is caused by an immunological or by a non-immunological mechanism. And while they are looking for that 'mechanism' they seem to be rather miffed that organisations, and some individuals, are willing to offer advice on how to diagnose and treat food intolerance with methods which have 'little scientific basis'.

This does not make sense. The medical profession have got to understand that parents who have a hyperactive child cruising around their ankles are desperate. In the real world, most parents will do almost anything that may help the child, even to contact organisations for nutritional advice which has 'no scientific basis'. Nor are the parents much interested in whether the child's inappropriate behaviour pattern improves using scientific evidence, non-scientific evidence or even anecdotal evidence. The same with some grown-ups. Many are getting fedup with suffering from continuous physical pain and/or mental disturbances to be prepared to wait umpteen years until the medical profession might one day find enough 'scientific evidence' to back up the curative powers of simple dietary changes and harmless nutritional supplements.

Some years ago Dr William Crook wrote an excellent letter to The Lancet about diet and childhood hyperactivity (133): "Sir, - In my general paediatric and allergy practice, I have found that 75% of my hyperactive patients improve, often dramatically, when their diets are changed. I base this statement on a clinical study of 182 hyperactive patients who came to me during a five year period (134). Sugar was identified by the parents as the leading troublemaker, with food dyes (especially red) and additives second. Many children also showed adverse reactions to a variety of other foods, including milk, corn, chocolate, wheat, egg and citrus fruits. Admittedly, this subject is emotionally charged and controversial, and several scientific studies of diet and hyperactivity have yielded doubtful or negative results".

"Moreover, the National Institute of Health consensus panel, to which your March 20 editorial refers, gave only lukewarm endorsement to the diet/hyperactivity connection. Before the conference I did a survey (135) of twelve paediatricians who were studying hyperactive children, using different defined diets which avoided not only food coloring and additives, but also other foods which commonly cause allergic symptoms in children (sugar, milk, chocolate, corn, wheat, egg and citrus fruits). The survey confirmed my clinical observation that over half of the food-sensitive, hyperactive children showed other typical signs and symptoms of systemic and nervous system allergy, including nasal congestion, dark shadows under the eyes, and pale colour in the absence of anaemia. Moreover, half of these children complained of headache, abdominal pain and muscle aching. This symptom complex was described by Randolph (136) in 1947 and again by Speer (137) in 1954, and has sometimes been labelled 'the allergy tension fatigue syndrome'."

"Naturally it would be helpful if the offending foods could be identified by immunological tests, including prick tests, radioallergosorbent assays, scratch tests, and leucocyte inhibition of histamine. However, the adverse reactions to foods which cause hyperactivity rarely belong to one of the four types of immunological reaction outlined by Gell and Coombs... In about 1745, James Lind observed that putting limes on board British ships prevented scurvy. Yet it was 50 years before supplementation of the diets of British sailors with limes and other fresh fruits and vegetables became a routine practice - and it was not until 1929 that Albert Szent-Gyorgi isolated vitamin C and provided the scientific explanation for the efficancy of limes."

"Hundreds of American physicians, including Randolph, Speer, and Rapp (136-138) have found that most irritable, unhappy, hyperactive children can be helped by a carefully designed trial diet in 5-10 days. And after the child's symptoms show a convincing improvement which lasts 48-hours, the food troublemakers can be identified by having the child eat them again, one food a day, over a second 7-10 day period. James Lind would have approved of this approach." (133).

The same Lancet edition published another letter by Dr Doris Rapp about the same subject (138): "Sir, On page 662 of your March issue you published an editorial on food additives and hyperactivity. When readers are given only a part of the evidence, it is difficult for them to help the many parents who ask if foods cause the changes they see in their children. In the past two decades, several physicians (140-143) have indicated that many foods, besides moulds, pollens and even chemical odours would alter their activity and behavior. The Feingold diet considers only artificial food colourings, flavours and natural salicylates. The subsequent dietary studies considered food colouring only".

"If a child has ten nails in his shoe, you can design the best double-blind study in the world, deleting one nail, but the child will still limp. You must use enough food colouring in a challenge study to produce symptoms. One child might need 2mg of dye, another 100mg. According to Swanson (144), the average child ingests 100-400mg of food colouring a day. The food industry subsidised studies used only 25mg per day in their double-blind challenge studies (145,146)"

"There are claims that a simple one-week diet eliminating accepted highly allergenic foods plus new modern suspects, sugar and food colouring, rapidly relieves symptoms in some affected children (138,143,147,148). Why cannot physicians recommend a simple diet composed solely of fruit, vegetables, and regular meats (no sausage, luncheon meats, and the like) for one week and then restore the questionable foods, one each day during the second week (i.e, milk, wheat, egg, sugar, dyes, corn and chocolate) and note the effect of each food? You may ask how to predict which patients may respond to diet. Look at them. If they have dark eye circles, bright read ears, and a glassy look when the Jekyll and Hyde behavior develops, the answer may be food. These children often have associated classical hayfever or asthma symptoms, headaches, abdominal complaints, leg aches, and behavior problems. The symptoms are often triggered by the very foods they crave..." (139).

Yet another letter by Vicky Colquhoun and Sally Bunday of the

Hyperctive Children's Support Group states the following (149): "Why the lack of treatment for hyperactive children? - Over the past years the Hyperactive Children's Support Group (HACSG) has been inundated with requests for help from thousands of exhausted parents, desperate for information and help, in an effort to reduce the disturbed behaviour of their children. The utter misery caused by such a child severely disrupts and damages family life. In addition to severe behaviour problems, sleeplessness, poor concentration, sudden mood changes, depression, compulsive touching and sometimes aggression, and other physical symptoms such as abnormal thirst, high pain threshold, sweating, bedwetting, ear infections, head, leg and tummy aches, asthma, eczema, repeated colds, coughs, and tonsillitis are all too often reported."

"We have found that many of these children have intolerances to foods, such as milk, wheat, sugar, chocolate, oranges, yeast and malt, food additives (colourings and preservatives). Tap water and pesticides also seem to be common problems, and often toxic metals such as aluminium figure in the cause of their symptoms. Deficiencies of important nutrients such as zinc, manganese, magnesium and vitamins have also been found in many children we deal with every day... For some children, simply removing coloured sweets, fizzy pop, chocolate and oranges is sufficient to bring about great improvements. Would that be too difficult to suggest as a start? If these hyperactive children do not receive appropriate treatment to overcome their problems, research and documented evidence suggests that they continue to display very disruptive behaviour, depression in many cases, and anti-social tendencies leading to quite severe social problems... Teenage hyperactives drink more alcohol than their friends. Chronic severe underachievement in school is a characteristic finding, despite high intelligence, and low self-esteem and a sense of failure are common..." (149).

Apart from this, Vicky Colquhoun and Sally Bunday have tried to tell the medical profession, already for years, that hyperactive children can improve, often dramatically, when given essential fatty acid supplements. Their findings were first published in 1981 (44). However, it took nearly fifteen years until the medical profession managed to find enough 'scientific evidence' to substantiate what Vicky and Sally had found all those years ago (45).

As seen, childhood hyperactivity can be treated simply and effectively by nutritional means (126-150). This being the case, it is quite incomprehensible to understand as to why ever increasing number of children suffering from hyperactivity are prescribed strong psychoactive medication such as Ritalin? What makes this practise particularly appalling is because Ritalin is associated with so many disturbing side-effects including nervousness, irritability, night terrors, euphoria, tremors, dizziness, dry mouth, sweating, palpitations, visual disturbances, dyskinesias and tics, rash, hair loss and growth retardation (151). Not only that but others have found that the drug is highly addictive, the withdrawal symptoms including severe clinical depression and suicidal tendencies (126). Even more frightening is that nobody seems to have the faintest idea how Ritalin, especially when taken long-term, can affect the child's brain which is still in its early stages of development.

Even so, according to the press: "More children given 'chemical cosh' (by Roger Dobson) Record numbers of children are being given the drug Ritalin to control their behaviour. Prescribing rates for the drug, which is used to calm hyperactive children, have trebled in the past year and are 24 times what they were six years ago. A study by a Southampton University researcher reveals that some children were given the drug four times a day for up to four years. Yet it found little evidence that the effects of the drug were monitored..." (152).

This shocking practise continues regadless that the latest research evidence shows that Ritalin has no beneficial effect on childrens' behaviour beyond seven to 18 weeks when it enforces submissiveness so that the child is more easily tolerated by everybody around him. Also, that the drug does not only fail to improve the child's learning ability, but that it impairs his thinking and mental function (153). Indeed, what a dreadful way to 'treat' a child! Have we no shame?

Not only that hyperactive children can be treated simply and effectively by dietary means, also childrens' intelligence improves by eating a nutritious diet and, if necesary, by taking additional nutritional supplements. This was proven by a carefully controlled double-blind experiment by Benton and Roberts (154). Another research experiment by Professor Eysenck and his team came to similar conclusions (155). Also, a recent press article reported that a junior school leapt up in league tables when it decided to ban the sale of crisps, fizzy drinks and sugary snacks in their tuck-shop and replacing them with fresh fruits. The idea came about when the teachers had noticed that after the children had been eating non-nutritious sugary snacks which were high in artificial food additives, they became very hyperactive and difficult to control. Soon after the junk was removed and replaced with fresh fruit, the childrens' concentration and learning ablity improved to the extent that the school's success rate in most academic subjects almost trebled (156).

Juvenile delinquency:
The most common mistake most doctors seem to make is thinking that hyperactive children will eventually 'grow out' of their hyperactive behaviour when they mature. This assumption is incorrect. Most follow-up studies on hyperactive children show that, even though they may be less hyperactive when they get older, they still continue being impulsive, excitable, distractable, restless and emotionally immature. An ever increasing number of research studies show that at least one third of the children diagnosed as hyperactive when young, end up as heavy drinkers and/or drug addicts (157,158). Other studies have found that about one quarter get involved in more serious crime (84,121,126,159).

According to Professor Bryce-Smith; "Follow-up studies of children originally diagnosed as hyperactive have shown, in comparison to controls, a higher drop-out and expulsion rate from schools, a higher rate of involvement in alcohol and drug abuse and a greater risk of coming before the courts... During a (voluntary) visit to a modern UK prison of young male adults convicted of serious crimes, I was informed by the prison psychiatrist that nearly all the inmates were hyperactive as children" (121).

The fact that an inadequate diet can lead to criminal behaviour has been proven over and over again. Some of the most convincing evidence comes from a series of studies conducted by an internationally known criminologist, Professor Stephen Schoenthaler of the Department of Social and Criminal Justice at California State University (160-164). His first two-year-double-blind experimental study among 276 juvenile delinquents held in a Virginia penal institute show that by eliminating only manufactured sugary junk foods and drinks and replacing them with fresh fruits, fruit juices and nutritious snacks, the incidence of assaults was reduced by 82%, theft was lowered by 77% and refusal-to- obey-an-order by 55% (160,161). The the same happened when he replaced a high sucrose diet with nutritious snacks in an Alabama juvenile institute (162).

His third experiment on diet and delinquency was conducted among 1382 juveniles that resided in three different Los Angeles County institutions. After the inmates' high sucrose diet was replaced with fresh fruits, fruit juices and nutritious snacks, the incidence of anti-social behaviour was reduced in all three by 44% (163). This study is particularly significant for two reasons. First of all, because the inmates' behaviour was observed while they were on a high and a low-sucrose diet. By literally acting as their own controls' eliminates the possibility that the control group would have been 'better behaved children' in the first place. Secondly, because the inmates' behaviour improved in all three institutions, this eliminates another possibility that one institute would have been more effective than another in dealing with young offenders (163). The same happened when Dr Schoenthaler tested his theory among 3,339 young offenders in a Northern California juvenile institute. After replacing junk foods with nutritious juices and snacks, the incidence of disruptive behaviour decreased by 42% (164).

Although these studies were designed largely to reduce an excessive sucrose consumption and thereby in preventing low blood sugar episodes (reactive hypoglycaemia), Professor Schoenthaler points out that the improvement in the inmates' behaviour cannot be placed on the reduction of sucrose alone. After all, as all fresh fruit contains vitamins and minerals needed for a well-functioning brain, this played a part. In addition, their behaviour improved by not eating manufactured snack-foods high in synthetic food additives that are also associated with mental health problems in susceptible individuals.

Another internationally known criminologist, Alexander Schauss came to similar conclusions (85,165,166). He points out that most acts of delinquency, vandalism and violence are largely spontaneous; performed without any fore-thought or planning. They involve a type of behaviour pattern which a well-nourished and non-toxic thinking brain would not even be interested in. These children, whose brains are simply incapable of thinking 'straight', do not commit crimes because they have been born bad but only because they feel bad. The main reason why so many youngsters feel bad is because their brains cannot work effectively due to the combination of the following: sub-clinical vitamin and mineral deficiencies, food and/or chemical allergies, low blood sugar episodes and/or an overload of toxic metals, particularly lead and/or cadmium. He believes that the only way these children can start behaving themselves is not to lock them up but to feed them with a nutritious diet and, when necessary, give them additional nutritional supplements.

The link between non-nutritious diet and juvenile delinquency was proven, yet again, by Barbara Reed, a probation officer. After she reviewed diets of thousands of probationers, she found that all had the same eating pattern in common: they did not eat any breakfast, they consumed high amounts of sugary foods and drinks and most hardly ever ate any fresh fruits, vegetables or good quality proteins. Her findings have been published in an excellent book entitled "Food, Teens and Behaviour" (167).

Most of the research evidence linking inadquate diet with juvenile delinquency comes from the United States. Now Britain has also decided to get into the act. This project, run by Bernard Gersh, a former probation officer, was designed to find out whether nutritional supplements are able to improve young offenders' behaviour pattern (168). Before the trial was due to begin I happened to meet Bernard Gersh in a London conference. So I decided to ask him why it is necessary to repeat these experiments in Britain as there is already plenty of research evidence from the United States which links non-nutritious diet with criminal behaviour? He agreed, adding, that it is neverthless necessary because until the same findings have been duplicated in Britain, the official opinion is that the American experiments have no value. Good grief! What is the matter with the 'official opinion'? Admittedly we speak English with different accents, but should this then automatically follow that British and American youngsters have different metabolic requirements?

Our justice system is currently going nowhere. All that is happening is that our youth crime is forever rising. According to a 1997 press report, young offenders are committing 13 crimes every minute, at a cost to the victims and the Government between £5-10 billion a year (169). These costs, however substancial, do not include the misery and fear that are impossible to verify. If we can reverse this trend doing nothing more drastic than by making sure that our youngsters are well fed, it must be surely worth a try? Instead of spending ever increasing amounts of money building more jails, institutions and correction facilities, we ought to spend it feeding our children with nutritious food. After all, no brain can be expected to show good judgement on a diet which contains hardly anything else but non-nutritious, additive-full junk.

Also, considering when Professor Bryce-Smith visited a prison for juvenile offenders he was informed that nearly all the inmates were hyperactive as children, it is therefore vital that we treat the condition before these children mature. Not by giving them 'chemical cosh' such as Ritalin to keep them quiet but treating them properly using effective dietary changes and harmless nutritional supplements (121-150). That way we are not only saving a tremendous amount in human and emotional resources but also ourselves a fortune in terms of special schooling, unemployment benefits, criminal justice system and building more secure institutions. This surely makes sense?

At the moment of writing, the government is proposing legislation that dietary supplements which have a 'physiological effect' on the body should be re-classified as medicines and, as such, they would require the same costly licence as pharmaceutical products which the health food industry cannot afford. This is really madness gone to the extreme. Particularly as official dietary surveys have repeatedly shown that the 'average British diet' is short of most vitamins and minerals needed to stay physically healthy and mentally alert (1-11). It looks as if the brains of our official mandarins are also so short of nutrients that they have lost the ability to think rationally.

Adult mental illness:
As with children, adult mental illness can be prevented, as well as treated, by nutritional means. For example, when Dr Vicky Rippere studied diets of several psychiatric patients she found that all had the same eating pattern in common. First of all, they did not eat any breakfast. If they did, it consisted of a couple of slices of white bread and several cups of sugary tea or coffee. Most ate hardly anything else for lunch but sugary snacks. The majority never ate any fresh fruits or vegetables. The main meal of the day consisted of manufactured convenience foods, usually eaten very late in the evening, when it was of the least use in providing energy for the day's activities (170).

Anyone who has been diagnosed as suffering from phobias or panic attacks, for example, should check whether these may be due to low blood sugar episodes. Similarly, if you have been diagnosed as suffering either from anxiety neurosis (171) or hyperventilation syndrome (172) because the symptoms of both are the same as associated with reactive hypoglycaemia (78,79,84).

Food intolerance in adults:
The symptoms of food intolerence in adults are varied. For example, physical symptoms are known to include: fluctuating weight, a persistent feeling of fatigue, palpitations, runny, itching or stuffed up nose,

sneezing, chronic cough, mild sore throat, itchy or blocked ears, swollen and painful joints, migraine headaches, bloated stomach, alternating constipation and diarrhoea, stiff and painful neck, rapid or slow pulse rate, weakness of limbs, excessive perspiration and flu-like symptoms. The most prominent mental symptoms associated with food intolerance are: a feeling of drowsiness, lethargy, depression, unresponsiveness, mental exhaustion and alternating dullness and irritability (84,173,174).

The late Dr Theron Randolph, one of the most respected pioneers on clinical ecology and nutritional medicine, places the mental symptoms associated with food intolerance under the heading 'brain fag', which describes well the most advanced form of this type of allergy (173). He points out that this condition is not easy to understand by those who have never experienced it. It is a form of debilitating mental fatigue characterised by a feeling of sadness, confusion, slowness of thought, depression, irritability, impaired memory, lack of comprehension, indecisiveness, mental lapses and speech difficulties. At times, these individuals feel so dreadful that they are quite unable to express their thoughts let alone concentrate on anything. The majority are never properly diagnosed even though they have thick medical files filled with a long list of symptoms largely mental in origin (173).

As the majority of the medical profession are not that keen on getting involved with patients suffering from food intolerance, it is not suprising that these patients are at best given some ill-defined diagnosis such as irritable bowel syndrome, fibromyalgia or similar. Another alternative is that they are told that their symptoms are 'all in the mind' and are therefore referred to see a psychiatrist. For example, an interesting study by Howard and Wessley, entitled "Psychiatry in the allergy clinic: the nature and management of patients with non-allergic symptoms" points out that yet another intriguing aspect regarding this type of 'non- immulogical' allergy is that its symptoms seem to overlap with other 'modern diseases' such as chronic fatigue syndrome (CFS), myalgic encephalomyelitis (ME), sick building syndrome, seasonal affective disorder (SID) and candida albicans (175).

According to the press, about a quarter of patients seeking treatment for bodily disorders have no physical disease but the their disease is all in 'the mind' (176). It looks as if nothing has changed during these past twenty years when the late Dr Richard Mackarness, another respected clinical ecologist, wrote these immortal words: "Like most general practitioners I had several patients crippled with illness for whose symptoms I was unable to find a cause. In the old days it was common practice to tell these people to pull themselves together and hope for the best. Nowadays these illnesses are more often labelled psychosomatic and the patient is offered psychiatric help, although this may amount eventually to being told to get on with it, in the nicest possible way of course, and with the prescription of tranquillising drugs... Because food and chemical allergy is not yet recognized for what it is, no statistical studies have been made, so we can only estimate the incidence of this type of illness as follows: 30% of people attending doctors' surgeries have symptoms exclusively traceable to food and chemical allergy, 30% have symptoms partially traceable to food and chemical allergy, and the remaining 40% have symptoms which are unrelated to allergy. My American colleagues give similar figures..." (174).

Yet another interesting point which connects allergies with mental health problems is that histamine, which is released in abundance during an allergy reaction, also acts in the brain as a neurotransmitter (177). Considering that many psychiatric medications, particularly those used to treat depression, such as tricyclics and related antidepressants such as imipramine (Tofranil) and amitriptyline (Lentizol and Tryptizol) inhibit the brain's histamine activity, indicates that particularly depression could be caused by underlying allergies (178). Some drugs used to treat psychoses seem to have similar action, particularly phenothiazine derivatives including chlorpromazine (Largactil), promazine (Sparine) and thioridazine (Melleril) (178,179). In short, considering that anti-histaminic medications are used in treating mental disorders, it is also likely that many mental health problems are indeed allergenic in origin (180).

A reason why so many doctors are still not familiar with nutritional medicine is largely due to the power of the pharmaceutical industy, but more about that subject later. For the same reason, most medical journals prefer to stay clear of the subject. For example, before the drug industry invented tranquillising medication in the early 1960s, reactive hypoglycaemia was mentioned frequently in medical journals as a cause for anxiety-related disorders and panic attacks (181-185). The same with food intolerance. Since the drug industry managed to come up with all kinds of potions to suppress symptoms associated with food intolerance, the medical press hardly ever mentions the subject. There are exeptions however, particularly The Lancet and the New England Journal of Medicine. In fact, I have based many findings in this book on articles published in The Lancet such as studies relating food intolerance with childhood hyperactivity (128,129,133,138). The Lancet has also published articles connecting food intolerace with migraines (186,187), rheumatoid arthritis (188) and irritable bowel syndrome (189). There are obviously thousands of others but these will suffice.

Schizophernia:

Of all the diagnosis concerning mental ill-health the label schizophrenia is probably the most feared. The same could be said about the treatment which, more often than not, consists of long-term use of psychotropic medications which are associated with a variety of disturbing side-effects. The latest idea is, however, that the diagnosis 'schizophrenia' should be abandoned and the treatment ought to concentrate on symptoms only.

Richard Bentall, Professor of Clinical Psychology of the Liverpool University, wrote an excellent article in The Times regarding the diagnosis and treatment of schizophrenia. He points out that even though vast sums of money and effort have been poured into schizophrenia research, yet the disease seems as baffling today as it was first described by Emil Kraepelin over hundred years ago. Every factor known to influence human behaviour has, at one time or another, been singled out as a possible cause. In the 1950s the chance discovery that chlorpromazine, the antihistamine drug, relieved the symptoms of some patients led to speculation that schizophrenia has biochemical basis. Many believed that abnormalities in parts of the brain containing the neurotransmitter dopamine might be responsible. However, no consistent support for this theory has been provided by subsequent studies. Some respond to neuroleptic drugs such as chlorpromazine, others benefit from lithium carbonate (the drug normally used to treat mania), and some fail to respond to any medication. The trouble is that all these drugs are associated with unpleasant side-effects. Unfortunately, because response to medication is unpredictable, psychiatrists sometimes increase the dose, producing severe side-effects without any benefits. Confusingly, most symptoms associated with schizophrenia also occur in other illnesses. Many experience schizophrenic symptoms such as hearing voices, but do not seek psychiatric help. "The time has surely come to abandon the diagnosis of schizophrenia altogether. It does not help clinicians to decide on treatment and it has misled researchers into lumping together people with very different symptoms. Research should focus on what patients actually complain of - hearing voices, feeling persecuted, difficulty in speaking. In the mean while, we should seek pragmatic ways to reduce the distress of patients and their families." (190).

One of the most prominent expert in the world in treating mental illnesses with nutrition is Dr Abram Hoffer (70,191,192). The Lancet published nearly forty years ago one of his double-blind research experiments which shows that schizophrenic symptoms can be cured, or at least much alleviated, by high doses of vitamin B3 (191). Besides vitamin B3 (niacin), he treats his patients with other nutritional supplements including vitamin C, B6, B12, folic acid and zinc. In addition, he found that many suffer from reactive hypoglycaemia and/or have severe food intolerances, particularly to wheat and/or dairy products. Furthermore, that urine of some individuals diagnosed as suffering from schizophrenia turned deep pink or mauve in colour when mixed with certain chemicals. This 'mauve factor' disappeared as soon as the patient became well. He named this condition malvaria (70,192).

71

Another of the world's foremost experts in psychochemistry, the late Dr Carl Pfeiffer, came up with similar findings. He also managed to identify that patients with this 'mauve factor' were secreting high amounts of a substance known as kryptopyrrole in their urine, thus calling the condition pyroluria which he treated successfully with vitamin B6 and zinc supplements. He estimated that about 30% of schizophrenics suffer from this condition (193). He found also that about 40% of individuals diagnosed as suffering from schizophrenia had high body copper and low body histamine levels. He named this condition histapenia which he treated with vitamin B3, B12, B5 (pantothenic acid), folic acid, zinc and manganese. Also, that about 20% of schizophrenics produce excessive amounts of histamine. He called this condition histaledia which he treated by supplementing the patients with calcium, zinc, manganese and methionine (an essential amino acid) (193).

Like Dr Hoffer, he noticed that many were suffering from reactive hypoglycaemia and/or severe food allergies, mainly to wheat and/or dairy products. Similarly, that most symptoms associated with schizophrenia can be cured, or at least much alleviated, by vitamin B3, B12, folic acid and zinc supplements. He also found that the following metabolic disorders can lead to symptoms associated with schizophrenia: heavy metal toxicity, drug intoxication, insufficient thyroid hormone secretion (hypothyroidism), wheat-gluten sensitivity and/or essential fatty acid deficiency (193). I already mentioned that Dr Horrobin and his team have found that some schizophrenias respond well to essential fatty acid supplements (41-43).

As seen, most 'schizophrenias' can be treated with nutritional means. The same goes for other mental health problems. For example, when Dr Hall and his team gave a thorough physical examination to a hundred psychiatric in- patients, they found that the majority were not 'mentally ill' at all but most were suffering from one, or a combination, of the following physical disorders which affected their mental state: sub-clinical malnutrition, folic acid deficiency, hypoglycaemia, allergies, anaemia, diabetes mellitus and an underactive or overactive thyroid function (194). In short, it looks that most mental illnesses are not 'mental' at all but physical in origin. This being the case, it is absolutely vital that before anyone is labelled as mentally ill, in whatever category, that the individuals are first examined as to whether their mental health problems are caused by underlying nutritional deficiencies and/or by other easily treatable physical disorders which are known to lead to a malfunctioning brain.

Senile dementia and Alzheimer's disease:
Even though the diagnoses differ, both share the same symptoms including a progressive impairment of memory, judgement and thought. The main differences between these two conditions is that senile dementia is thought to be a natural occurence in old age whereas Alzheimer's disease is considered as a specific clinical condition affecting individuals at any age, though becoming more prevalent among the elderly. The other difference is that the decline of intellect in senile dementia is fairly slow compared to Alzheimer's where the deterioration is quite rapid. Whether a person had suffered from senile dementia or Alzheimer's disease can only be determined by examining the brain structure at post mortem. The most noticeable pathological features associated with Alzheimer's are neurofibrillary tangles within the brain cell fibres and the presence of 'senile plagues' on the brain's structure (192).

Alzheimer's disease:
The cause of Alzheimer's disease is still unkown. However, some research evidence is linking the development of Alzheimer's with excessive aluminium contamination (195,196). As aluminium cannot easily by-pass the blood-brain barrier, researchers have concentrated on the blood-brain barrier itself. When experimenting with rats, it was found that when they were placed on a low-zinc diet, this led their blood- brain barrier to become 'leaky' which allowed aluminium to infiltrate into the brains quite easily (197). As a result, it is suggested that one reason for developing Alzheimer's may be a low dietary zinc intake which, after years, could make the person's blood-brain barrier

so 'porous' that it allows aluminium, and other toxic metals, to be deposited into the brain structure (198).

The latest contribution to the development of research into Alzheimer's was made in 1998 by The Oxford Project to Investigate Memory and Ageing (OPTIMA). The study consisted of 250 volunteers suspected of suffering from the early stages of Alzheimer's and 100 healthy elderly controls. The project lasted for several years, during which time the researchers were able to gather a great deal of information from the participants including regular brain scans, blood samples and vitamin-B measurements. Also, before the project began, participants had consented to having their brains examined on their death so that the results could be compared with the laboratory findings (199).

As the result, it was found that the ones who were positively diagnosed as suffering from Alzheimer's, had folic acid levels 30% lower than the controls. Because folic acid is one of the nutrients required for reducing high homocysteine levels, the researchers wanted to find out whether the Alzheimer's disease victims had higher homocysteine levels compared to the control subjects. The results show that those with high homocysteine had three times the risk of developing Alzheimer's disease compared to those with normal or low levels (199).

Homocysteine derives from methionine which is an essential amino acid. Unlike methionine which is an antioxidant, homocysteine is a powerful oxidant and thereby able to initiate lipid peroxidation and free radical damage. High homocysteine levels have already been associated with the development of heart disease (54) and now, with Alzheimer's. However, folic acid is not the only vitamin required for remethylation homocysteine, others are equally important, particularly vitamin B12 (cobalamin) and B6 (pyridoxine) (200).

Senile dementia:
Unlike Alzheimer's which is a specific disease process, senile dementia is considered as being a part of the natural ageing process. This assumption is incorrect. Even though getting old is inevitable, becoming senile is not. According to Dr Hoffer, senility can be prevented,

even reversed, by eating a diet which contains, besides antioxidant nutrients, all the vitamins, minerals and essential fatty acids needed for a well functioning brain. In addition, all highly processed manufactured convenience foods should be avoided. Not only because they are low in nutritional value but also because most contain high amounts of sucrose, trans-fatty acids and synthetic food additives which are harmful for health (192). In other words, the diet to prevent senility is the same as that required for preventing other degenerative conditions such as heart disease, cancer and mental illnesses.

Even though there is no substitute for a nutritious diet, Dr Hoffer points out that in many cases diet alone may not be able to provide all the essential nutrients needed to reverse a failing memory and mind. In fact, he has found vitamin B3 (niacin) supplements particularly beneficial because the vitamin participates in a number of biochemical reactions including electron transport and oxidising reducing processes and, as such, it has the ability to improve blood circulation, neurotransmission and energy production. An additional benefit with niacin is that it is the safest 'medicine' for lowering harmful LDL-cholesterol whilst elevating the useful HDL-cholesterol levels (192).

The most insidious reason for developing senile dementia results from taking prescribed medications. According to Dr Millard, doctors do their patients an injustice if they believe that a failing memory is always a sign of old age as many drugs are associated with a reduced mental function, including both the short and the long acting benzodiazepines, antihistamines, digoxin, barbiturates, diuretics, tricyclic antidepressants and indomethacin (201). The same with cimetidine, benzhexol and the anti-Parkinsonian drug, levodopa (202). Even the long-term intake of naproxen and ibuprofen have been associated with memory loss (203). This being the case, in situations where a patient complains of a loss of memory, the first question a doctor got to ask is whether anything he has prescribed might be the cause? In fact, according to Dr Millard, it is surprising that the medicated elderly pass any mental tests at all (201).

All synthetic medications are considered by the body as toxins.

Therefore, once digested, the body's first reaction is to detoxify the offending substances immediately. This process is ezymatic, requiring antioxidant nutrients (204). In cases where the person's vitamin and minerals reserves are already low, it is obvious that this drug elimination process will reduce them even further, leading eventually to an excessive accumulation of drug residues and hence to ever increasing side-effects. To prevent this, anybody on multi-medication should make sure that their antioxidant intake is sufficient for the detoxifying process. If in doubt, it is sensible to take a balanced vitamin and mineral supplement every day.

CHAPTER 4

THE PESTICIDE POLLUTION PROBLEM

The fear that the human race has been poisoning itself by its own ingenuity was first commented on in the 1960s by Rachel Carson in her book "Silent Spring" which predicted the dangers of pesticide pollution (205). Nothing has changed since her chilling book was published, though ever accumulating scientific evidence shows that our modern agricultural practices are not only destroying our planet but also our precious health and reproductive capacity.

The modern agricultural industry sprays every year literally billions of gallons of highly toxic insecticides, herbicides and fungicides on our food crops. It is estimated that cereal crops receive approximately 5-8 applications per growing season, while for high-value crops such as vegetables and fruit, 10-15 applications are normal. In addition, during storage, most cereals, fruit and vegetables are dosed again with pesticides to protect them against storage diseases. This post-harvest application is performed using a so-called 'bucket and shovel' method when pesticides are mixed with freshly harvested products and just thrown on top of the already 'treated' crops. As a result, even though the actual harvest may have been relatively uncontaminated, this crude post-harvest storage treatment can add a considerable amount of pesticides to the produce destined for sale (206). Furthermore, thousands of tons of pesticides are sprayed each year around railway embankments, canals and waterways to remove excess weeds. The same with our parks and other recreation areas. They are also added to many manufactured products including wallpaper pastes, wooden furniture, DIY products, carpets, natural-fibre textiles and so on and so forth (206).

The modern agricultural industry also uses pesticides as 'animal medicines' such as sheep dips, warblefly, lice and mange treatments as well as to control flies and other insects in livestock houses. Even some of our own medicines contain pesticides. For example, warfarin which is used for killing rodents, is prescribed to humans because it possesses an anticoagulant action and is therefore able to prevent the formation of blood clots. Also shampoos designed to kill human head lice contain pesticides (206). The toxic ingredients of pesticides fall into many chemical categories of which the most widely used are organochlorines (OCs) and organophosphates (OPs).

Organochlorines (OCs):
Pesticides that contain OCs include DDT, lindane, dieldrin and aldrin. The pest-destroying action of OCs is to disrupt and jumble nerve signals leading to paralysis and death. Because OCs are practically non-biodegradable, persisting in the environment for decades, they are highly dangerous for the whole ecosystem. In addition, having a particular affinity to fatty tissues, they are able to transfer through the food chain from one species to another, from the smallest of insects all the way to large mammals including humans. It is therefore not suprising that DDT and its break-down products have been detected in the fatty tissues of most people tested (206).

Xeno-oestrogens:
Ever increasing research evidence is linking foetal exposure to OCs, particularly DDT, with a decline in male fertility and other hormone-related disorders (207,208). The reason why these chemicals are particularly hazardous to the unborn child is because they mimick the action

78

of the female hormone, oestrogen. Besides DDT, other man-made chemicals have been associated as having an oestrogen-mimicking activity, particularly those connected with the plastics' industry. To date, at least the following chemicals have been found to be responsible: bisphenol-A, phthalates, octylphenols, nonylphenols and poly-chlorinated biphenyls (PCBs). Bisphenol-A is used in the manufacture of polycarbonate of which most plastic containers, bottles and similar packaging are made. Phthalates, on the other hand, are used to make plastics more flexible and nonylphenols are added to polistyrene and PVC products to make them less breakable. Polychlorinated biphenyls (PCBs), having a high resistance to heat, are used in circuit breakers, electric switches, voltage regulators and as coolants in electric transformers. Also dioxin which is a highly toxic by-product formed by pulp, paper and bleaching industries are known to have oestrogen-like action. Similar compounds are used in the manufacture of some toileteries and even spermicide foams. In fact, most man- made chemicals, ranging from pesticides to paint additives are currently under suspicion. All these chemicals that are known to possess oestrogen-mimicking activity are now collectively known as xeno-oestrogens (208).

The reason why these chemicals are particularly hazardous to the unborn male is because the human foetus always starts life as female. A number of hormonal cues, which begin to take place in the very earliest weeks of foetal growth and development, have to occur at the right time to orchestrate the events which determine whether the child will be born male or female. If it is to become a male, at about six weeks, the male hormones trigger a series of events which instruct the growth of the male reproductive tract whilst female ducts begins to regress and are eventually re-absorbed (208).

This process of masculinization requires the presence of Sertoli cells which are responsible for the formation of the male sexual organs including sperm and testosterone production. The reason why these xeno-oestrogens are able to damage the male sexual identity is because they have an ability to suppress the multiplication and action of these vital Sertoli cells in the womb, consequently hindering the chromosomal differentiation and masculinization process (208).

Ever increasing research evidence is also linking early foetal exposure to these oestrogen-mimicking chemicals in males with clearly noticeable birth malformations including undescented testes and other genital deformities. Others have found that foetal exposure to these xeno-oestrogens, in both males and females, can eventually result in the development of hormonal-triggered cancers, such as cancer of the breast in females and prostate and testicular cancers in males, which only reach their pathological state in adulthood when they come under additional hormonal influences (208).

According to a well-referenced book by Deborah Cadbury entitled "Our Sterile Future" (208), these hormone-disrupting chemicals have been found to be resspossible for the following; Firstly, they can lead to structural changes obvious to the naked eye at birth such as reproductive organ malformations. Secondly, they can produce permanent changes in the foetal brain growth and development which can be expressed in later life as a reduced intellectual capacity. Thirdly, they can produce delayed effects, only visible under microscope, such as changes in cell structure and growth leading eventually to cancer formation. And finally, at a more fundamental level, they can alter the genetic code (DNA) in such a way that cells lose their ability to express themselves as nature intended leading to both hormonal and reproductive complications (208).

Professor Niels Skakkebaek, of the University of Copenhagen, was the first one to observe that in the past fifty years human sperm counts had fallen by 50%. Since then, other researchers have come to similar conclusions. In fact, it has been estimated that male sperm counts are falling by something like two per cent a year. Besides that, there has been a significant fall in sperm motility and the percentage of normal sperm. Others have found that the number of couples seeking treatment for infertility has increased considerably in the past twenty years. For example in Britain, one in six couples are known to suffer from infertility problems. Although these have been traditionally viewed as a female problem, the latest findings indicate that in about 40% of cases it is the male partner who is responsible (208). Besides male infertility, foetal exposure to DDT and other xeno-oestrogens have been associated, at least in animal species with 'homosexuality'. Whether this also applies to humans it is just anybody's quess. If nothing alse, at least these chemicals have been found to have a considerable 'feminizing effect' on the male (209).

The most alarming thought is that our modern world is practically surrounded by these xeno-oestrogens. They are not only found in the foods we eat but also in our detergents, paints, water pipes, bottle caps, childrens' toys, electric gadgets, toiletries, spermicide foams, clothes and shoes. In other words, we do not only eat them but sit on them, have a bath in them, walk in them, drive in them and even make love in them. In fact, one just can not think of any 20th century activity which would not be contaminated one way or another by these oestrogen-mimicking substances.

Though ever increasing evidence has demonstrated the dangers associated with these 'gender-bending' chemicals, it looks that multinational chemical manufacturers are determined to continue using them until governments outline a comprehensive stragedy forcing them to switch to less harmful materials. Governments, on the other hand, don't seem to be prepared to do anything of the sort until scientists can give them definite proof of how dangerous these chemicals really are. Considering that most 'scientific' research is funded by the industries, it is naive even to imagine that any findings from that source would conflict with the vested interests. One cannot help wondering sometimes what kind of people are those who are in charge of these multinational chemical corporations? One would have thought that one day they also would like to procreate and carry on their genes. And when they do, one would also assume that it is just as important to them, as it is to us, that the offspring they produce is born as healthy and well-balanced as possible.

Organophosphates (OPs):
From the mid-1970s, when persistent OCs were reduced from the

agrochemical market, they were replaced by highly toxic, but biode-gradable organophosphorus (OP) pesticides. The toxic pedigree of OPs was established during the Second World War when scientists were looking for potent nerve gases for military purposes. Virtually all types of OPs depress acetylcholinesterase activity, leading to an excessive acetylcholine output, nerve paralysis and death (206).

Most of the evidence on the adverse health effects of OP- exposure relates to accidental occupational poisoning. The World Health Organisation estimates that there are at least three million acute cases of unintended pesticide poisoning worlwide, including about 28,000 deaths (206). Others believe that the death toll could be as high as 40,000 a year (210). However, acute pesticide poisoning in the Western World is a fairly rare incident, unlike chronic pesticide exposure which seems to be an every day occurence. In fact, given today's extensive use of pesticides during food production, it is almost impossible for anyone to avoid a cocktail of pesticide residues (206,211,212). A recent official survey by the government's Pesticide Safety Directorate (PSD) found that 25% of foods analysed contained pesticide residues, 1.4% exceeding the 'maximum residue limits' which can put consumers' health at risk. However, this was believed to be a substantial underestimate because when researchers sent further food samples which were purposely 'spiked' with over a hundred pesticide residues to three different research laboratories for analysis, the results showed that all three had underestimated the pesticide levels by more than 20%. (212).

Ever accumulating research evidence is linking a long-term, low-level exposure to OPs with a variety of neurotoxic and neurobehavioural effects which have been particularly noticeable among farmers who have been dipping sheep. During the dipping, the sheep are immersed in a tank that contains a liquid with high levels of OPs to protect the animals against parasites such as scab and blowfly. Annual sheep dipping was compulsory until 1992, when it became voluntary. Even though farmers are advised to wear protective over-clothing, they are still known to become affected. The symptoms of low- level OP-exposure include: depression, aggression, memory lapses, blurred vision, chronic fatigue, aching limbs and joints, difficulties with co-ordination, muscle weakness and suicidal tendencies (206,213).

Furthermore, numerous studies have found a high incidence of cancers and related disorders in individuals that have been occupationally exposed to low-levels of pesticides. These are now known to include prostate and breast cancers, leukemia and non-Hodkin's lymphoma (206,213,214). Similarly, with delayed neurotoxicity. Consequently, ever increasing number of epidemiological surveys have linked chronic pesticide exposure to the development of Parkinson's diseases, multiple sclerosis and motor neurone disease. Also with the development of allergies and other immuno-regulatory disorders such as chronic fatigue syndrome (CFS) and myalgic encephalomyelitis (ME) (215).

Another worrying aspect of chronic low-level pesticide contamination is their ability to cause birth defects. For example, when the London Food Commission conducted a thorough toxicological survey on active ingredients currently permitted to be used by UK pesticide manufacturers, they found that of 426 chemicals listed, 68 were carcinogenic (cancer producing), 61 were mutagenic (affecting the genetic code) and a further 35 had teratogenic (ability to cause birth malformations) properties (211). The mutagenic action of pesticides became particularly noticeable when American servicemen who were exposed during the Vietnam war to a defoliant called Agent Orange, fathered infants with an unusually high number of birth defects (206). Similar problems are now found to occur with some children born to Gulf War veterans.

Gulf War Syndrome:
Literally thousands of British and American servicemen and women who went to the Gulf are claiming that the effects of the war has left them suffering from a wide variety of ill- effects, including aching and swelling joints, memory loss, dizziness, headache, blurred vision, chronic fatigue, skin disorders, shortness of breath, panic attacks and so on. Some are claiming that the Gulf service has left them permanently

crippled with more serious conditions such as kidney failure, epilepsy, cancer, blood disorders and motor neurone disease. This cluster of illnesses is now known universally as the Gulf War syndrome.

It is still not known what is the cause for this Gulf War syndrome, but ever increasing research evidence is pointing to an excessive exposure to OPs which were sprayed in abundance on military tents to protect the troops against a plague of disease-carrying flies and other bugs (216,217). The troops were not only exposed to OPs, but to many other toxic chemicals. For example, they were given NAPS tablets (nerve agent pre-treatment sets) to counter against possible chemical attack. They were also vaccinated against diseases such as botulism and bubonic plaque, some receiving simultaneously as many as nine different innoculations in one day. In addition, they were vaccinated against anthrax poisoning. As the anthrax vaccine on its own would have taken months to become effective, to accelerate its protective qualities, these anti-anthrax innoculations were combined with petrussis (whooping cough) vaccine.

Considering the toxic cocktail of chemicals these veterans were subjected to, it is not suprising at all that many became ill. However, it is a complete waste of time in trying to figure out which particular chemical might have been responsible because, according to the basics in toxicology, the effect of any given chemical should never be looked at in isolation. After all, most of us tend to be able to tolerate the effect of one toxic chemical alone, but the same cannot be quaranteed when exposed simultaneously to a cocktail of chemicals as the synergistic (combined) effect can potentiate one another so that the combination can become even lethal (218).

It looks that this was indeed the case with the Gulf War syndrome. This was confirmed at the Duke University Medical Centre when scientists wanted to find out which particular chemical might have been responsible for making the Gulf War veterans ill. The results show that when test animals were exposed to just one chemical these Gulf War veterans were subjected to, it did them no harm. However, when they received the combination of the chemicals, this led to a powerful nervous system damage (219,220).

A reason why some veterans fell ill when exposed to this cocktail of chemicals and others didn't, was because the enzymatic capacity between individuals to deal with chemical toxins varies. The ones who were able to tolerate the effect obviously had a well functioning detoxifying metabolism and a good immune system function, both of which depend, besides on hereditary factors, also on a nutritious diet.

Mad Cow Disease (BSE):

Let's move from the Gulf War to the 'Beef War' which left millions of animal corpses on the battlefield. Whilst the bodies of the cattle have been incinerated, the actual 'Beef War' was fought in Brussels between the British government and the European Union. This 'war' began in the mid-1980s when British cattle suddenly started to stagger and fall all over the place. These poor creatures were eventually diagnosed as suffering from BSE (Bovine Spongiform Encephalopathy), popularly known as Mad Cow Disease. Further research established a similarity between BSE and a human disease known as CJD (Creutzfeldt-Jacob Disease). Finally it was decided that the development of CJD in humans arises by eating BSE-infected cattle which in turn resulted in our European partners refusing to see any British cattle, mad or otherwise, on their shores.

CJD is an extremely rare form of progressive human brain disease (encephalopathy), affecting about one person in a million. It takes years to develop but when it manifests itself, it leads rapidly to a complete neurological break- down, dementia and death. Due to the long incubation period, CJD is mostly found in the elderly. The basic aetiology for encephalopathies is still not fully understood but they are thought to be caused by an aberrant form of small protein fractions called prions which act as a degredable and inter-changable signalling mechanism during neurotransmission. It is believed that both in CJD and BSE, some prions start to fold up the wrong way. In this form they begin to act like a template, persuading others to do the same, which eventually leads to a formation of insoluble plagues on the brain structure and further to BSE and similar encephalopathies.

Since eating BSE infected cattle was first linked to the possible development of CJD in humans, the course of the disease has changed somewhat. Instead of affecting the elderly, the victims have become younger and the period of the infection shorter. Also, when the brains of these younger victims have been examined at post-mortem and compared with samples taken from older victims, the disease pattern was found to be different. Instead of the infected areas being small and regular, the brains of the younger victims show more random and considerably larger destructed areas. These findings indicate that there could be two different forms of the disease. It is not yet known whether this 'new variant' CJD, which to date has lead to about 80 human deaths, is a new disease or whether it is a mutation of the original one. Likewise, no one knows as yet whether this new version has been around for a long time but has never been adequately diagnosed. Furthermore, there is still no proof whether eating BSE-infected cattle is the actual cause for this 'new variant' CJD. Be as it may, ever since eating BSE infected cattle was connected with the possible development of CJD, the story has hardly been out of the headlines. Not only guestioning whether BSE can cause CJD, but also what has caused BSE in the first place. Some believe that BSE was caused by feeding scrapie-infected sheep remains to herbivoreous bovines whilst others are in the opinion that it was caused by feeding them protein pellets made out of their own relatives.

However, the latest theory is that BSE is nothing to do with 'contaminated feed' but the condition is caused by being exposed to organophosphate pesticides. This was suggested by Mark Purdey, an organic farmer, with long-term research interests into the causation of BSE (215). When the first cases of BSE were reported, Purdey was already sceptical that infected feed could be the cause because there had been no cases of BSE in any animal born and bred on organic farms even though some of these herds had also been fed unwittingly with the supposedly 'infected feed' before the official ban.

Purdey noticed that the symptoms of BSE such as nervousness and unco-ordinated movements paralleled to those of chronic OP-poisoning. This in turn led him to conduct a thorough overall survey of BSE cases in Britain when he found a significantly higher number of BSE cases in areas where an organophosphate, namely Phosmet, had been used as a warble fly treatment (215). Also, that Britain was the only country in the world to have enforced routine use of Phosmet at such high levels. However, the ministry refused to give any credence to his claims that BSE could be caused by organophosphate poisoning until experiments at the Institute of Psychiatry found that Phosmet can indeed induce abnormal movement and distribution of prion proteins inside living cells (221). Since the emergence of this startling laboratory evidence, Purdey's findings are now finally taken seriously (222).

Another reason why 'contaminated feed' just cannot be responsible for the development of BSE is because even after the suspected feed was banned in 1989, it did not lead to the eradication of BSE. In fact, since the ban, literally thousands of new BSE cases have been detected among British herds. Also, before the feed was singled out as the possible cause, Britain exported literally thousands of tons of the same stuff abroad (223). Considering that cattle all over the world has been masticating the same 'contaminated feed' we have been giving to our cows, BSE became only rampant in Britain.

However, it could be argued that just as with Gulf War syndrome, it is feasible that the BSE epidemic in Britain could be caused by a combination of factors. After all, over and above the warble fly treatment, most of our intensively- reared animals are subjected to many other pesticide residues such as those used to control the spreading of flies and other insects in their tightly packed animal houses. As well as this, they are given all kinds of antibiotics in the name of 'preventive medicine' and another lot of the same as 'growth promoters'. In fact, considering the amount of toxic chemicals our cattle are exposed to, it would not be suprising if the 'contaminated feed' may have also played a part. Let's face it, if an animal is fed with not much else than dry pellets made from other animal debris, it not suprising that their resistance against toxic insults is practically nil. After all, just as with humans, all warm- blooded mammals need to be well fed and watered to possess the necessary enzymatic activity required to deal with different kinds of poisons.

This also explains why no cases of BSE have ever been recorded among cattle reared on organic farms. Not only are these animals fed a highly nourishing diet, but they are kept in a natural and toxin-free environment. Considering the seriousness of this BSE-saga, it is difficult to comprehend why the fact that organically reared animals were not affected was just ignored? All that happened was that everybody blamed somebody else for this BSE catastrophy. The public blamed the farmers for subjecting their animals to cannibalism. The farmers blamed the animal feed companies for selling them 'contaminated feed' whilst the feed manufacturers blamed the government for allowing them to use all sorts of 'contaminated' animals bits in their food manufacturing process.

Finally the government decided in their infinite wisdom to get rid of the whole problem by resorting to mass slaughter. This in turn resulted in farmers being heart-broken because they were forced to cull perfectly healthy cattle whilst abattoirs and rendering plants were in turmoil because they did not have the capacity to deal with this 'eradication' process effectively. To add to misery, the whole folly had to be paid by a taxpayer which amounted to about £4 billion which was divided to compensate dairy and beef farmers for the financial hardship forced upon them and to pay abattoirs and rendering plants for culling and incinerating the 'infected' herds. Some money was also allocated to pacify the beef exporters and livestock auctioneers to help them get back on their feet.

However, one of the most disturbing aspects of this massive slaughter was that it was not much to do with the actual 'eradication' of BSE but the whole performance was aimed at pacifying the European Union so that they would allow our beef products back into Europe. This is madness in the extreme. When our EU partners demand that we have to turn the British countryside into a bovine charnel house, we oblige. Even worse. It didn't make any difference how many cattle corpses we offered on the EU altar, our partners were still not prepared to allow British beef, however healthy, into their already over-saturated beef markets. If the EU policy is motivated by hysteria that can only be pacified by mass slaughter there is no knowing where it will all end. One cannot imagine a better illustration of the level to which the present Common Agricultural Policy (CAP) has sunk. Some say that repatriating agricultural policy to British control could be worse. Is it possible?

Whilst this blood letting went on, research grants were allocated left right and centre for further 'scientific research' in trying to establish whether eating BSE infected cattle could really be a cause of CJD. Every thinking person can see that this is not only a waste of scarce resources but also a waste of time because, as with all diseases with a lengthy incubation period such as encephalopathies, the results can never be clear-cut and definite. Besides studying and comparing clusters of epidemiological factors, all scientists can do is work on probabilities and guess the rest. Though the unfortunate victims of the 'new variant' CJD were fairly young, it is unlikely that it can ever be catagorically proven that their demise was really caused by eating BSE infected meat.

One of the most stupid ideas was to start feeding BSE- infected cattle tissue to chimpanzees to see whether our nearest relatives may also succumb to CJD. Before any results would emerge, it was estimated that the animals had to be fed BSE-contaminated cattle remains for at least ten years. Good grief! What on earth is the justification for force-feeding chimpanzees, who rather prefer to be vegeterians, BSE infected meat when the whole British island is already teeming with closely related human species who have been eating the stuff for years? All the 'scientists' have got to do is sit tight, observe, and at worst, start counting!

Not only have taxpayers already paid billions for the compensations caused by this BSE catastrophy, literally millions were spent on a so-called 'BSE inquiry' (224). One wonders whether this will ever end? Instead of spending never-ending sums on BSE/CJD research which is bound to tell us nothing more than what we already know and further millions for the 'BSE enquiry', the government ought to channel the money to support organic farming. Not only are we putting our own health and reproductive capacity at risk with intensive farming methods, they also have been responsible for most food- related crises such as salmonella in eggs and now, this BSE- catastrophy.

The most cruel aspect of factory farming is that it has turned our defensless fellow creatures into mere objects of large scale meat production i.e. the more animals can be packed into less space, the more profit to the farmer and the cheaper the meat to the consumer. Considering the tightly packed conditions in which these animals are forced to exist their short and miserable lives, it is not suprising that if an infection is present, it spreads like wild-fire. As a precaution, these poor creatures are literally doused with antibiotics. In addition, they are given another hefty dose of the same as 'growth promoters'. In fact, it has been estimated that at least three fifths of all antibiotics are used to 'treat' animals rather than human beings. Also, that more than a tenth of the antibiotics are administered to promote faster growth rather than to cure diseases caused by intensive farming methods (225).

Conclusive evidence shows already that this inscriminate antibiotic use among livestock has led to the emergence of antibiotic-resistant 'super bugs' capable of infecting human beings. The latest findings indicate that antibiotics thought of as a last resort against severe cases of typhoid fever, paratyphoid, salmonella and E.coli poisoning were at risk of being rendered ineffective because related antibiotics were being used in agriculture (226).

The modern agricultural industry seems to carry nothing but bad news. Whilst contaminating our food, driving our cows and sheep farmers mad and creating an ever increasing army of antibiotic-resistant 'super bugs', it has also poisoned our drinking water supplies. For example, when Friends of the Earth conducted a drinking water quality survey on 298 British water supplies, it found that 76 per cent of the supplies tested were contaminated with up to sixteen different pesticide residues (227). Yet another problem associated with modern agriculture is the ever increasing use of nitrogen-based fertilizers of which only about half is taken up by the crop, the other half being lost in a variety of ways such as leaching into our ground water reservoirs. In fact, it has been estimated that about 1,000,000 British households are consuming water exceeding the official EC Maximum Residue Levels of nitrogen and, if no action is taken, this figure could rise by the early part of the next century to as high as 4,600,000 households (227). Even though nitrogen is a natural element found in all plant, soil, water, animal and human matter, this indiscriminate use of inorganic nitrogen can do us a great deal of harm. For example, after combining with the amines in our body chemistry, it is converted to nitrosamines which are known to be one of the most powerful cancer-producing substances (206,228). Besides, crops that have been grown using inorganic nitrogen, are nutritionally speaking of a very poor quality. They consist of an abundance of green foliage whilst are practically void of most essential vitamins and minerals (229). By pushing quantity rather than quality, most foods produced by modern intensive agriculture are very low in nutritional value. As the result, they are also partly responsible for the development of cancers, heart diseases and other degenerative conditions (230).

There is no question whatseover that in order to restore our health, sanity and reproductive capability, we have to move from intensive farming methods to organic farming. The latter does not only produce high-quality and nutritious food, but it rears healthy animal stock without cruelty whilst, at the same time protecting our precious and fragile environment. If we really want to alter the way how our food is produced, changes will only emerge if there is a sufficient public pressure to warrant them. The pesticide-laden produce and contaminated animal bits will soon disappear from our supermarket shelves if we stop bying them. After all, like any other business, supermarkets are there for profit motives only and if they realise that their goods do not sell, they will soon do something about it.

Admittedly organic produce is currently more expensive than the industrialised variety. However, as industrial food prices are forever rising due to the ever increasing expenses associated with the Common

Agricultural Policy (CAP), even this will soon be a myth. For example, it is estimated that each family in Britain is paying, on average, about £1,000 a year in higher taxes and food bills to subsidise the Common Agricultural Policy (CAP) which is used, besides paying direct grants to farmers, to storage surplus production so that food prices can be kept artificially high (231).

Escalating food prices affect all of us but obviously the poorest section of society is hit the hardest because they spend a bigger proportion of their income on food. It really is high time to re-examine the European Common Agriculture Policy (CAP) because, in its present form, it is a highly expensive, food-destroying disaster. For example, not that long ago it was estimated that nearly three million tonnes of fruit and vegetables including apples, peaches, nectarines and cauliflowers were destroyed to keep prices artificially high (232).

Despite much-trumpeted reforms associated recently with the EU farm policy, nothing has really changed. Consumers are still paying a high price for a system that is not only failing farmers and damaging our health and economics but also destroying our precious environment. What is more ironic is that first we are forced to subsidise farmers to grow all these food mountains using highly toxic chemicals and then we are also expected to pay for the consequent damage. The 'hidden' costs associated with conventional factory farming were highlighted well in a letter to the press by Craig Sams: "Sir, Michael Hornsby's report of July 29 on Britain's abysmal incentives to organic farmers included the usual superficial price comparison of organic food versus conventional produce. The real costs of conventional food is not found on the supermarket till receipts but is hidden in water bills, tax bills and healthcare costs. One billion pounds have been invested by water companies in clean-up equipment, along with an annual £121 million water-cleaning cost to remove pesticides and nitrates from the water, so that it can meet EU minimum standards. The soaring level of food poisoning, with 93,000 reported cases in 1996 compared to 19,000 in 1985, is the cost to the National Health Service, not to the purchaser of factory-farmed meat. The common agricultural policy costs every UK household £20 per week. In 1983 organic farmers banned the feeding practices that led to BSE, a cost to the nation most recently estimated at £4 billion, and still rising. Poisoning by pesticides is an occupational hazard for farm workers, particularly those who handle sheep dip. The NHS picks up the treatment cost, but the real cost is the waste of human potential. Genetic engineering of food, an attemp to industrialise the fundamental processes of nature, holds risk that only experience will enable to assess. If all these costs were diverted to the supermarket bill then market forces would do the rest." (233).

There is yet another, most interesting point, which favours organic farming. That is; if we are not prepared to alter our ways, the time may not be far off that the whole world is populated by organic farmers only because they seem to have far healthier sperm compared to other mortals. For example, not that long ago, a Danish study found that organic farmers had 100 million sperm per millimeter of semen, compared with an average of 54 million among the others, and 227 live sperm per million sperm against the average 181 (234). If nothing else, this study indicates that the fall in male fertility in the last 50 years could indeed be caused partly by being exposed to pesticide residues.

Genetically Modified (GM) Foods:

Only a few words about genetically modified (GM) crops which are creeping onto our plates whether we like it or not. Unlike natural cross-breeding which only takes place between species which are closely related, genetic engineering involves a random insertion of genes to the host, not only from completely unrelated plants but also from animals, viruses and bacteria. To make tomatoes and strawberries frost-resistant for example, the technique allows the transfer an 'anti-freeze' gene from an arctic fish. To find out whether the desired gene has been tranferred successfully into its new host, the technique uses 'marker genes' which are believed to be antibiotic-resistant. No wonder consumers are getting pretty fedup with the whole performance. Not only because they are expected to eat all sorts of strange viruses, bacteria and antibiotic-resistant genes with their tomato ketchup but vegans are simply horrified that they are forced to swallow their strawberries with fish genes tucked inside.

Considering that genetic engineering is only at the most primitive stage involving processes which are not only random but very much 'trial and error', there is no way of telling how these GM foods will affect our health in the long term.

In the mean while, doctors are to be enlisted to watch any links between eating genetically modified foods and rise in birth defects, cancer, arthritis and diabetes. Also, ministers, acting on advice from the Government's chief medical and scientific advisers, are planning to establish a national surveillance system to discover wheter consuming GM foods may trigger new patterns of heart diseases, allergies, asthma and other degenerative conditions (235).

However, by far the most worrying aspect concerning these gene-altered crops is their impact on the environment as no one knows what will happen when they begin to cross-pollinate with their closely related wild species. To prevent this, GM crops are separated from others by 'buffer zones' which are no more than about 200 meters wide. All well and good except the official mandarins had obviously forgotten bees which have no respect for boundaries whilst searching for their daily provisions (236).

Whilst we are waiting to see how these 'Frankenstein foods' will affect our health and what will happen when GM crops begin to cross-pollinate with their wild relations, results from field tests have already found a highly significant premature death rate and reduced fertility among beneficial ladybirds who ate greenfly (aphids) fed on genetically modified potatoes. Also that these crops are killing our butterfly population (237).

There is no question whatsoever that if we are not prepared to take notice of these early warnings the silent spring, which Rachel Carson predicted in 1962, will be well and truly silent. According to Nick Nuttall, genetically altered plants could wreak environmental havoc; "It is the year 2020 and the most silent of silent springs, apart from the rustle of genetically engineered oil-seed rape, wheat, maize and other 'designer' crops nodding in the breeze. Songbirds such as lark, linnet and thrush, long in decline, have finally fled the English countryside because the seed- producing weeds on which they depend have been eradicated from fields and hedgerows by relentless chemical spraying made possible by biotechnology. Meanwhile the hum of bees and other insects has also been silenced, thanks to the planting of genetically altered crops that produce insect-resistant toxins. They annihilate not only aphids and other pests but also beneficial insects on which birds and bats depend..." (238).

Similar sentiment was expressed by Geoffrey Gray: "Sir, about 45 year ago I had to fix a mesh screen to my study window to keep out moths, butterflies and other insects. Birdsong filled the air by day and owls could be heard at night with other sounds of animal activity constantly present. Today I have no need to erect an insect-proof screen and the only birds around are seabirds and the toughest of survivors, such as pigeons. Mr Roy Helmore (letter, May 22) wants a panel of scientists unadulterated by hoi polloi to reassure him about agricultural policies. Would this be the same panel of scientists that has encouraged the use of hormones and antibiotics in their dairy industry? Would it be the same scientific community that has advocated the use of pesticides and herbicides which has resulted in the destruction of many species of insects and the extinction of uncountable numbers of birds and animals? And all to what purpose? So that we can benefit of 15-year-old meat in refrigeration, butter mountains and other iniquites practised by avaricious food manufacturers? I believe planting of GM crops in the open environment is extremely hazardous, and the idea that any sane person would trust the scientists, eminent or otherwise - especially at the behest of the Ministry of Agriculture - is almost beyond belief. There is an ancient wisdom that says as the world's species diminish, so does the survival of the mankind. We were given the responsibility of looking after the world and we have made a singularly bad job of it." (239).

CHAPTER 5

THE AIR POLLUTION PROBLEM

Although practically invisible, air pollution contains a cocktail of toxic chemicals which do not only make us ill but also kill. The worst culprit that churns out these insidious toxins is our beloved motor car. Our modern industrialised world is also practically cocooned in an unseen envelope of electromagnetic pollution and low-level radiation which poses danger to our health. Let's concentrate first on traffic congestion which is responsible for the following pollutants:

1) **Carbon monoxide** which is a waste product of fuel combustion. When it enters the blood stream it has an ability to deprive the body of oxygen. At higher concentrations it kills, but at lower concentrations it causes headaches, drowsiness and slowing of mental and physical reactions.

2) **Nitric oxides** which are readily oxidised to nitrogen dioxides and nitric acid which irritate lungs, thereby worsening asthma, bronchitis and other respiratory disorders.

3) **Ozone** which is formed at gound level when nitrogen oxides and hydrocarbons react with sunlight forming a photochemical smog. In this form it is able to travel across vast areas, picking up fresh injections whilst moving from one dense traffic spot to another. Subsequently, high ozone levels are not only found in

cities, but in suburban and rural areas. At lower levels, ozone irritates the mucuous membranes of the nose, mouth, throat and lungs, aggrevating asthma and leading to breathing difficulties. At higher leves it is known to damage lung tissue and to reduce the immune system function.

4) **Sulphur dioxide** which is formed when fossil fuels are burned. Power stations generate the worst sulphur dioxide emissions but also cars are responsible. Once in the air, it is converted into sulphuric acid which irritates the eyes and leads to breathing difficulties.

5) **Particulates** which are formed when diesel fuels are burned. They consist of tiny flecks of invisible ultra fine particles which contain a cocktail of toxic chemicals including sulphates, polyaromatic hydrocarbons and nitrates which have both carcinogenic (cancer producing) and mutagenic (damaging the genetic code) properties. Because particulates are minute, they are able to penetrate deeply into the lung tissue, aggrevating asthma and bronchitis as well as causing severe breathing difficulties.

6) **Benzene** which has been added to unleaded petrol to replace lead to make it burn more smoothly. It is a cumulative toxin which has both carcinogenic and mutagenic properties (240).

Benzene derives largely from cars driven without catalytic converters. The most worrying aspect of this 'green fuel' is that it needs comparatively high amounts of this poisonous chemical before having any effect, thereby making this 'environmentally friendly' fuel equally, if not more dangerous than the leaded variety (241). This is yet another classic example of introducing hasty legislation ahead of adequate scientific knowledge. All that we have done is to exhange lead which attacks childrens' brains and intellect to a poisonous substance that causes cancer and birth defects. Even catalysts are not as brilliant as first thought because their use has now been linked with increasing ground ozone levels (242).

Another blunder that has emerged on the motoring front is the diesel engine which was potrayed years ago as a virtuous alternative to petrol driven vechicles. However, the latest studies indicate that the ultra fine particles arising from diesel fuel are responsible for all sorts of health problems including lung and heart diseases, and that the number of deaths attributable to diesel pollution may range from 2,000 to 10,000 a year (243).

Official surveys have shown that at least 19 million Britons a year are exposed to air pollution levels in excess of international guidelines. Also that asthma is increasig at an alarming rate: there are now three million recorded sufferers and that one in seven children is affected. Ever increasing research evidence has connected asthma with air pollution (244). Also thousands of heart attacks a year have been associated with traffic pollution. One of the most comprehensive studies made on the subject found a clear link between air pollution and one in 50 heart attack patients treated in London hospitals which is equivalent to 6,000 cases (245). Furthermore, it has been found that polluted air may be responsible for between 12,000 and 24,000 emergency hospital admissions a year among people with chest conditions. Similarly, that it may contribute to the death of up to 24,000 frail and elderly people a year (246).

One of the most detailed investigation on the link between air pollution and health was conducted in the United States. The results show that cities with high pollution levels had death rates up to 26 per cent higher than less polluted ones. The consistency of the findings across the surveyed cities were remarkable. It was found that the death rates from lung cancer and heart disease were more strongly associated with high pollution levels than deaths from respiratory diseases such as asthma and bronchitis. Further investigations revealed that the pollution levels in the American cities with the highest death rates was similar to that found in London, Birmingham, Newcastle and Cardiff (247).

In short, at least from our health point of view, our beloved motor car has turned out to be one of our worst enemies. Not only can it maime and kill by direct impact but it also fills up doctors' surgeries and hospital waiting rooms with patients that have been poisoned by its highly toxic effluent. Not only that, but this misery is costing us already a fortune. According to some estimates, traffic pollution is costing Britain more than £50 billion a year in healthcare costs. Also that premature deaths due to the same have reached 6,000 people a year, double the deaths from traffic accidents (248).

It looks as if we are suffering now from a brand new disease which could be diagnosed as car-addiction. Besides ruining our health, economics and environment, it has also been responsible for changing our lives out of all proportion. Before this disease became widely spread, our little towns and villages were vibrant and pleasant places to live in because they had many colourful little shops where people were able to buy their daily provisions. Ever since we have allowed our four-wheeled coffins to dominate our lives, one shop after another has been closed and boarded up due to lack of support. It is really heart-breaking to see how the once, ever so lively towns and village centres, have gradually become only fit for vermin to live in. Because most local shops have ceased trading and the nearest shopping facilities are miles out of town, the ones who do not have a car are really in trouble. The older generation seems to be particularly affected because even many post offices, from where senior citizens used to collect their pensions, have moved into some far-away, out-of-town shopping complex. In other words, today's world is not designed for legs but for wheels only.

The great irony of this ever increasing car-dependency is that the more people take to their cars, the greater part of their lives is spent sitting inside their motor vechicles coughing, wheezing, spluttering, choking and scratching, whilst going nowhere. In fact, today's traffic congestion is already so bad that the so called 'freedom of having a car' amounts to not much else but freedom to choose one's traffic jam. Even more ironic is that it is the motorist who seems to suffer the most. Not only is he forced to squat a considerable chunk of his life in traffic jams but he is literally poisoning himself in the process.

So who is to blame for this ever increasing traffic chaos? Motorists obviously blame other motorists for not having enough sense to leave their cars at home. Others blame the lack of an easily affordable intergrated transport system. Some blame the oil industry for not selling cleaner fuels which are available in other countries including in the United States and Scandinavia. Not only is the quality of petrol there cleaner, but they are only allowed to use City Diesel which has nearly half the particulate emissions compared to the type sold in Britain. Admittedly, some British petrol stations sell City Diesel but the outlets are very few and far between. So why are cleaner fuels not more easily available in Britain?

According to a television documentary which ivestigated the dangers of traffic pollution on health, when the interviewer asked one of the oil industries' representatives why the British consumer cannot buy similar, minimally polluting fuels to those available on the continent, he replied that it is not the oil industry's responsibility to set fuel policy standards in Britain but the government's. Adding, as soon as the government sets an appropriate legislation for cleaner fuel policy, the industry will obviously oblige. After this, the interviewer asked the minister of transport why the government hasn't legislated a cleaner fuel policy? His reply was that the only reason why the government has decided against it is because less polluting fuels are more expensive and the British motorist will find it quite unaccepatable. As usual, when the government acts incompetently, we have only ourselves to blame. In this instance, the government considers that the only reason we are content to poison ourselves and our children with the dirtiest fuels available is because we are too mean to do otherwise.

In the meanwhile, one way to reduce ever-increasing traffic pollution is to curb private cars entering large town and city centres. There is already overwhelming evidence that city centres from which cars are banned, have a far higher retail turn-over, more prosperity and generally a far better quality of life compared to cities which are congested with traffic. Similarly, it would help if more freight was transported by train instead of by lorry. It would also be a good idea if every school could use small buses to transport children back and forth from school, or parents were able to organise an efficient car-share system. In cases where the distance to school is relatively short, at least from the children's health point of view, allowing them to walk to school and back is an excellent idea because physical inactivity during childhood is associated with different kinds of health problems in later life. If parents are too nervous to allow their child to walk alone, several children could walk together as there is always safety in numbers. Or parents could share the responsibility of walking a group of children to school and back.

Even though there are ways of sanitising the car by means of modern technology, the positive aspects of less polluting vehicles will soon be overtaken by the sheer number of ever increasing car ownership. Besides creating unthinkable traffic chaos, the pollution will still be there. An excellent letter to The Times by Dr Robin Russell Jones, sums up the whole situation 'Sir, The Times deserves congratulations on its timely investigation into the adverse effects of air pollution on human health. Your readers should also be aware, however, that environmental groups have been making precisely these points over the last decade. I quote from the submission which I prepared in 1984 on behalf of the Friends of the Earth to a House of Lords select committee on the EC directive regarding air pollution by motor vehicles: Carbon monoxide, oxides of nitrogen, ozone and hydrocarbon emissions all pose a threat to human health. In particular, the substances known as polycyclic aromatic hydrocarbons contain a number of carcinogens which have been implicated as the agents responsible for the higher incidence of cancer observed in urban areas. A recent American study concluded that from 11-21 per cent of current lung cancer can be attributed to air pollution. The mutagenic properties of exhaust emissions have been measured in Sweden, showing that diesel emissions were ten times more mutagenic than petrol emissions. The latter, in turn, were ten times more mutagenic than emissions from an engine running on unleaded petrol and fitted with three way catalytic converter. By the year 2025 the Department of Transport predicts an increase in traffic volume of between 80 per cent and 140 per cent. Instead of blundering on with its massive road-building programmes would it not be more sensible to create an intergrated transport policy on both environmental and health grounds?' (249).

Indeed, the only conceivable way to reduce our ever- increasing car-dependency is that the government organises an easily affordable intergrated transport system. This is certainly not going to be easy because since British Rail and the bus services became fragmented due to privatisation, not only have prices increased out of all proportion, but the public are completely at a loss as to which train or bus takes them where, what way, how and when? Directly due to scanty information, uncordinated timetables and baffling connections provided by priva-tised bus and rail industries, ever increasing number of people are abandoning the idea of travelling on public transport (250). Even passengers attempting the simplest of journeys are getting fedup be-cause fares are so expensive. As I do not drive a car, I rely either on my bicycle or public transport. Luckily I live in a place where transport is easily accessible but because fares are increasing all the time, the time will not be far off that it would be cheaper to own a car. There is no question whatsoever that an integrated transport policy is a brilliant idea but it is quite useless if we cannot affort to use it.

Though most air pollution is caused by traffic congestion, industries are also to blame. Maybe one of the most widely spread pollutants created by industry are sulphur dioxide emissions which result from power stations burning fossil fuels. Once in the air, it forms sulphuric acid which is the main component of acid rain which does not only harm our health but also creates a great deal of havoc wherever it falls. Besides damaging buildings, it kills huge forests and contaminates water ways poisoning marine life in the process. As air is no respecter of boundaries, one country tends to blame another for these catastrophies. The same with carbon dioxide emissions which are responsible for global warming. Whilst temperatures are forever rising and Antarctic ice is literally melting in front of our eyes, all that is happening is meetings are held all over the world trying to decide which country is mostly responsible.

Not only are our cars and factories making us ill, our modern industrialised world is literally enveloped in unseen environmental hazards that can harm us in a variety of ways. Radioactive discharges from nuclear processing plants have, already for years, been associated with all kinds of health problems including cancers and birth defects. The same with electromagnetic pollution coming from high voltage power lines. Also, televisions, radios, computers, microwave ovens, mobile telephones and similar electrical appliances are known to do us harm.

The dangers associated with mobile phones have only very recently become the focus of media attention. For example, the latest research evidence is linking the use of mobile phones with the development of cancer and Alzheimer's disease (251). Others believe that asthma and other allergy-related disorders are made many times worse when the person is exposed to microwave frequences coming from mobile phones, computers, televisions and similar gadgets (252). Also VDU radiation from computer screens is associated with health problems including depression, excessive fatigue, runny nose, itchy eyes and short-term memory loss. (253).

Most official surveys claim that the mechanism by which air pollution causes ill health is not fully understood. This is not suprising because most laboratory experiments have concentrated on the effect of one pollutant alone instead on the mixture of them. Just as with the Gulf War syndrome, it is a complete waste of time in trying to figure out which particular pollutant is resposible for making us ill, it is the combination of chemicals we ought worry about. For example, when independent research groups in Britain and abroad examined research studies concerning the adverse effects air pollution, pesticide residues and contaminated food/water supplies on human health, it was found that this chemical cocktail was not only responsible for literally thousands of human deaths a year but millions were suffering from all manner or mental and physical health problems because of it (254).

There we are then. Whether we like it or not but one of the reasons why our hospital beds are full and our doctors are rushed off their feet is because we have traded our precious health with modern technology. This is rather a Faustian paradox as there is no way that we can have both. We simply got to accept the indisputable fact that if we wish to surround our lives with all sorts of comforting gadgets, we also have to accept that we will always be suffering from more cancers, heart diseases, respiratory illnesses, asthma, allergies, infertility and mental health problems. As we cannot turn the clock back, it is up to us, as individuals, to make at least some effort in trying to reduce our ever-increasing environmental pollution. For example, we can do ourselves, our future generation and our precious planet the greatest of favours by simply learning to walk again and by supporting organic farming.

CHAPTER 6

THE PHARMACEUTICAL INDUSTRY

Those who like to argue that we can only thank modern medicine that our life expectancy has risen in the last hundred years overlook the fact that up to the first few decades of the twentieth century infant mortality rates were extremely high. In Britain, for example, the death rates among babies under one year old has fallen since the beginning of this century by more than 85%. When these massive child mortality figures are taken out of the equation the average life expectancy in the developed countries has most certainly not risen in the way we are led to believe (255).

It is also worth noting that modern medicine had nothing to do with the decrease in child mortality statistics, as these were almost entirely a result of better living conditions, particularly sanitation. We cannot even thank the vaccination programmes for an increased life expectancy since epidemiological studies have shown that mortality rates for infectious diseases as varied as cholera, typhoid and whooping cough fell, also as a result of better sanitary conditions, to a fraction to their former levels, long before vaccines were even invented (255).

Despite enormous amounts of money spent on Western health- care, we seem to be nowadays sicker than ever before. In Britain, for example, where free access to doctors and hospitals is available to everyone, life expectancy for the 40-year-olds is only decreasing. What's more, even though Americans spend, on average, around 12-14% of their cross national income on high-technology medicine, they seem to be sicker and die youger than individuals living in less 'doctored' countries (255). Most prematured deaths are caused today by cancer or heart disease. Even those who manage to survive these biggest 'killers', many are spending their lives suffering from some chronic disability or another. If we are not plagued by arthritis, diabetes, asthma or allergy, we are suffering from depression, anxiety, panic attacks or what ever else.

What these chronic non-infectious diseases have in common is that most can be prevented, even reversed, by consuming a wholesome diet and by avoiding excess exposure to toxic pollutants. Another thing these diseases have in common is that modern medicines cannot really cure any of them, only to suppress the symptoms. The trouble with this kind of 'treatment' is that it allows the underlying disease process to fester uninterrupted and, in time, make the condition even more chronic and irreversible. The modern pharmaceutical industry obviously wants us to believe otherwise. By deploying a highly sophisticated mixture of hard science and hard sell, they have managed to convince almost everyone that 'pills mean health'.

Drugs have always been around us ever since cavemen collected herbs. Until the end of the nineteeth century most drugs were still plant-derived herbal remedies. Besides herbs, earlier physicians also used all sorts of strange nostrums as 'medicines' such as animal dung, powdered mummies, sawdust, lizard's blood, dried vipers, frog sperm, crab's eyes and other such weird things (256). In addition, as late as the nineteenth century, bleeding, purging, puking and perspiring were still used as standard medical treatment (257). Pondering this grim array of elixirs and prodecures which were medically respectable in their day, it is sometimes difficult to comprehend how the physicians managed to maintain their position of honour and respect throughout medical history? Another thing that comes to mind is that the human race seems to be clearly distinguishable from other species by its willingness to put up with all kinds of physical insults and to consume anything, however distasteful and appalling, as long it believes that it is 'good for health' (257).

The pharmaceutical industry, as we know it today, started only in the latter part of the nineteenth century when the first pill-making machine was invented. It began to expand when scientists were able to establish chemical make-ups of some herbal remedies. From these advances came aspirin for example, which is a synthesised version of a herbal medicine derived from willow tree bark. However, it took until the mid-20th century before the drug industry really got going. The reason for this sudden expansion can be directly attributed to the development of antibiotics. First came the sulphonamides followed soon by the penicillins (257). From then on, something like euphoria set in.

The modern pharmaceutical industry is now a colossal money-making enterprise. At one end are organic chemists, biochemists, biophysicists and pharmacologists deploying all conceivable parapher-nalia of science to develop and test new compounds. At the other end is the promotional part consisting of drug representatives and massive advertising campaigns. Even though the industry likes us to believe that it exists only for the sake of mankind this is not so. The pharma-ceutical industry, just like any other successful industry, exists for profit motives only. This being the case, the industry also prefers to manufacture drugs which will offer them a long-term profit margin. They are particularly keen on manufacturing drugs which, in order to offer the desired relief, have to be taken regularly, preferably several times a day. Because so many are now suffering from some chronic disability or another, the industry is literally booming.

To date, the industry has managed to manufacture pills and potions for practically every conceivable condition. They have anti-arrythmias, anti-hypertensives, anti-depressants, anti-convulsives, drugs for ul-cers, diuretics, drugs for lowering cholesterol, bronchodilators, pain-killers, tranquillisers, sleeping pills, pills for controlling pregnancy and for replacing hormones, ointments for suppressing acne, eczema and what ever else. In addition, the industry has stacked pharmacies with a vast array of over-the-counter (OTC) medication that can suppress coughs, colds, aches, snuffles, pimples and spots. The list is endless!

People are never more vulnerable than when they are ill, or think they are ill. In fact, it has been estimated that between 50-80% of adults in the industrial world are taking at least one pharmaceutical drug every day (258). In Britain, for example, and 'average' citizen takes at least three types of prescription drugs and five different OTC- medications every year (214). This massive drug-taking is certainly a goldmine for the pharmaceutical industry but unfortunately not so good for our health. Not only because modern medications cannot cure chronic disease conditions but also because most drugs, especially when taken long-term, can do us more harm than good.

Most people tend to imagine that a drug is like an arrow which zooms directly to the wanted target whether it is meant to ease a pain in the hip or to reduce mental anxiety. This assumption is incorrect. Contrary to this, the action of most drugs is non-specific which means that the medicines we take do not only affect the target organ but act inscriminately throughout the whole body chemistry. This unselective drug action is also why most drugs have unwanted side-effects (151). Another reason why medicines can make us ill is because they are made of synthetic chemicals which our body 'sees' as toxins. Therefore, once digested, the body's first reaction is to begin to detoxify the offending substance immediately. The human body can detoxify some drugs faster than others. This is known in pharmacology as a half-life which defines how long, on average, it takes half of the drug to be eliminated from the body. As this detoxifying process is enzymatic, needing not only antioxidant nutrients, but also other vitamins and minerals, it is obvious that in individuals whose vitamin and mineral reserves are low, the drug residues begin to accumulate leading gradually to over-toxification and thereby to ever increasing side-effects (204).

In fact, it has been estimated that two out of five people receiving clinical drugs experience side-effects that are in many instances far more serious than the condition being treated (259, 260). Those who are on multi-medication have to be especially careful because the accumulation of one drug into the body chemistry may not do too much harm but the same cannot be quaranteed if his body gets over-saturated by a cocktail of drug residues.

No-one really knows how many are injured by prescribed medication. This is partly because drug injury is still largely a hidden problem, grossly under-reported, hard to detect and often impossible to verify. Rough estimates of the annual incidence of adverse drug reactions (ADR) are based on different methods but most of the following samples are derived using a variety of industrial and government sources. Assuming that 10% of all ADRs are recognised and reported, the number of hospitalisations in Britain that are believed to be wholly, or at least partly due to drug side- effects, is estimated at about 240,000 cases each year (259). Direct deaths caused by prescribed medication in the United Kingdom are difficult to estimate but the figure is thought to be somewhere in the region of 15,000 deaths per year which is over double the deaths caused by road accidents (260).

The situation seems to be equally alarming in the United States. For example, when researchers examined the results of 39 studies of adverse drug reactions, it was estimated that they were affecting as many as 2.2 million hospital patients a year, leading to 106,000 deaths (261).

These findings are a good example of the fact that even though medicines are 'legal' drugs they can be just as dangerous as 'illegal' ones whether one thinks of heroin, morphine or arsenic. Not only that, but some prescribed medications are as addictive as street drugs which became particularly noticeable with tranquillising medication (benzodiazepines).

Since the introduction of the first benzodiazepines in the early 1960s, they have become the most widely prescribed medicines in the world. They are not only used as anxiolytics (tranquillisers) and sedatives (sleeping pills), but also as anti-convulsants (treating certain types of epilepsy) and amnestics (to relax patients before surgery). However, most are prescribed either as tranquillisers or sleeping pills.

A notable difference between these two is their half-life but even so, both still carry the same risk of dependency and lead to similar symptoms on withdrawal (259).

Side-effects associated with a regular use of benzodiazepines are known to include the following: excessive sedation, lack of co-ordination, shaking, muscle weakness, dry mouth, double or dimmed vision, vertigo, giddiness, mental confusion, disorientation, poor concentration and memory, speech impairment, feeling of unreality, emotional anaesthesia, agitation, anxiety, panic attacks and agoraphobia. These symptoms develop insidiously whilst the patient continues taking the therapeutic doses, increasing with dosage reduction and becoming especially troublesome during withdrawal (84, 262, 263).

In fact, the withdrawal symptoms associated with a long-term benzodiazepine use can be extremely disturbing. Besides the symptoms above which are experienced in far more intensive form, they also include: chronic insomnia, acute sensitivity to sound, light touch and smell, persistent headache, seizures, chest and muscle pains, stiff and painful neck, tremors, nausea, vomiting, hyperactivity, severe depression and anxiety, hallucinations, agitation, aggression, paranoid and schizoid episodes, panic attacks and extremely disabling phobias, particularly agoraphobia (84, 262, 263).

The average withdrawal period is estimated as being approximately six weeks for each year the individual has been taking the therapeutic doses. Furthermore, some researchers have found that a long-term benzodiazepine use can be responsible for a loss of memory in a way that whatever a person had learned, or experienced, while on the medication, he will have great difficulty in remembering after the withdrawal period is over (84). Others have come up with findings that long-term benzodiazepine use can lead to noticeable cerebral ventricular enlargements and hence to a reduction of brain size (264).

It is sometimes difficult to figure out where one should draw the line as far as drug addictions are concerned. Take a fairly recent benzodiazepine litigation scandal for example, where 5,000 plaintiffs tried to sue the pharmaceutical industry for their addictions to tranquillising medication which literally ruined their lives. Nothing came of it, only the legal profession pocketed enormous fees which the taxpayer had to pay. What seemed likely to be the biggest personal injury action in British legal history collapsed at a cost of 30 million pounds to the taxpayer. Not a penny was recovered for any of the plaintiffs after six years of battling. The claims collapsed after the Legal Aid Board's decision to withdraw funding because of 'the difficulty of establishing liability' (265).

So there we are then. As far as this massive drug addiction scandal was concerned there were no penalties to the manufacturers nor to the suppliers. The only penalty was put upon the consumer. Not only did he have to pay to obtain the drug in the first place, he also had to pay for the legal costs when trying to sue the industry which manufactured such a dangerous product. One might have thought that the pharmaceutical industry should have been held at least partly responsible. On the other hand, if the industry was not aware that their product was both highly addictive and able cause so many distressing side-effects, this is even worse. In fact, whichever way one looks at this situation regarding the side-effects associated with any given medication, it seems to be nothing but an unscrupulous swindle because, if anything goes wrong with the medicines we take, nobody else is responsible but the poor consumer who did not have enough sense to stay clear of the dangerous product in the first place.

Since the thalidomide disaster when thousands of women gave birth to malformed infants, drug companies were asked to provide increasingly rigorous safety and efficacy standards concerning their products to which they claim to comply. When a drug is first developed in the test tube it is tested for toxicity using animal experiments. Next, it is tested on healthy human volunteers and finally on a group of patients suffering from a complaint the drug is expected to treat (266). Considering that our medicines have gone through the most stringent and detailed battery of safety tests, why it is that dangerous medications are still filtering into the consumer market?

Reasons may be many but without a doubt the main one is because the inital testing for toxicity is performed by using animal experiments. Leaving aside all sentiments such as why so many millions of innocent furry creatures must suffer and die for the sake of humanity and looking at vivisection purely from a scientific point of view, testing drugs on animals that are destined for human consumption is an utter waste of time because animal metabolism cannot be compared with human metabolism. Not only are there great differences in overall structure but also between the composition and size of most bodily organs. Also, the basic biochemistry and enzymatic activity can differ a great deal between human and animal species. This is why animals hardly ever respond to toxic substances in the same way as humans do and vice versa.

For example: morphine sedates humans but stimulates cats; aspirin causes birth defects in rats and mice but not in humans; penicillin acts as an antibiotic for humans but is poisonous to guinea pigs and hamsters; insulin can produce deformities in laboratory animals but not in people; arsenic kills humans but is harmless to guinea pigs, chickens and monkeys; digitalis raises blood pressure in dogs but lowers it in humans; botulin is dangerous to both humans and mice but cats just thrive on it (255, 267).

Furthermore, animals seem to be able to detoxify drug residues at a faster rate than humans. Take an anti- inflammatory drug such as phenylbutazone for example, which has been responsible for an estimated 10,000 human deaths worldwide. When the drug was tested on rhesus monkeys they were able to detoxify the drug residues in eight hours, dogs and rats managed to do it in six and rabbits in three. But when the same drug was given to humans, it was found that they needed up to 72 hours to detoxify the drug residues (267-269). No wonder that phenylbutazone passed animal experiments with flying colours whilst killing thousands of people.

Yet another reason why animal experiments can be misleading is because the drug is tested for its toxicity on perfectly healthy and well fed animals whereas, in the real world, the same drug will be consumed by humans who are either frail, elderly or not well at all. Also, unlike laboratory animals who are exposed to only one drug at a time, many sick humans are taking a cocktail of different medications and it is the combination of drugs we have to be wary of.

In short, using animal experiments for testing drugs destined for human consumption is not only highly unscientific but positively misleading. They do not only cause untold suffering for animals but at the same time they allow the pharmaceutical industry to manufacture dangerous medications which do not only make us ill but also kill. If for no other reason than to save our own skins and sanity we have simply got to stop degrading and dehumanising ourselves with this vile animal butchery!

As we live in the world of highly sophisticated technology, there are already many, truly scientific methods, with which drugs can be tested without the use of live animals. For example, they can be tested using human tissue cells 'in vitro' (267, 268). Also, modern technologies such as cromatography and mass spectrometry offer an excellent opportunity to separate drug substances at their molecular level to identify their properties (267, 270). Furthermore, quantum pharmacology and modern robot-controlled chemical synthesis offer an excellent tool for studying the molecular structure of chemicals (271). In addition, the Ames test can be used in conjunction with 'in vitro' tests to determine whether a substance may have either teratogenic or carcinogenic properties (267, 272).

An international body of doctors who have been protesting, already for years, against the futility of animal experiments, states the following: "Results from animal tests are not transferable between species, and therefore cannot guarantee product safety for humans. In reality these tests do not provide protection for consumers from unsafe products but rather are used to protect corporations from legal liability" (273). This says it all. The only reason why the pharmaceutical industry uses live animals for testing their drugs for toxicity is not to protect the consumer but only to protect the industry from any liability that may arise if we get harmed by taking their medications.

According to Dr Vernon Coleman, vivisection is without doubt the most vital key to the success of the drug industry because, whatever the results, the industry cannot lose. If an experiment shows that a drug is harmless when fed to animals, the industry labels the drug as safe for human consumption. If, on the other hand, experiments show that a drug causes serious problems when fed to animals, these results are dismissed by the industry on the grounds that animal experiments cannot be regarded as relevant to humans because of the enormous anatomical and physiological differences (255).

By using this double-edged absurbity the pharmaceutical industry continually launches new drugs for human consumption which are found to lead to most serious problems when given to animals. In his book "Betrayal of Trust", Coleman lists names, and detailed information provided by drug companies, of over 50 different medications currently in use which were found to cause cancer and other serious problems when fed to animals. He also lists names of 85 thoroughly tested medications which passed animal tests with flying colours but neverthless had to be withdrawn from human consumption because they were found to cause serious side-effects in humans, some fatal (255).

In his book, published in 1994, Coleman also mentions tamoxifen which, even though it was found to cause liver tumours when fed to rats, was neverthless hailed by the pnarmaceutical industry as one of the greatest 'wonder drugs' in the prevention and treatment of breast cancer (255). However, the latest research findings indicate that after taking the drug for two years, the number of women developing cancer of the womb lining doubles and after five years it quadruples compared with women not taking it (274). Here we are again. Due to differences in overall structure, basic biochemistry, enzymatic activity and composition of most bodily organs, tamoxifen causes liver tumours in rats and cancer of the womb in human species.

The drug industry seems to exhibit an almost obsessional urgency to sell their medications. In their rush to the marketplace, the companies have persistently been caught exaggerating the beneficial claims of their drugs whilst minimizing the dangers. Also, in the hope of placing their products in the best possible light, they are known to use many unscrupulous tactics. For example, they choose most carefully who will test their medications. By so doing, it would be naive to think that they do not try to select those 'experts' who are likely to give them the most favourable report. Also, because they are paying for the experiments, they can determine the trial design so that if a drug has an apparent weakness they will arrange it to be tested in ways that are less likely to reveal the flaws. Equally, they are able to cancel any trials that may turn out to be a threat concerning their products. Even in cases where clinical trials have been conducted fairly but when the results are not quite as 'satisfactory' as expected, the industry can still continue to exercise censorship by choosing to publish the positive results only while ignoring the negative ones (266).

Some might wonder why drug industries behave so unethically? The simplest answer is that it could be extremely expensive to behave well. After all, as literally billions of pounds are riding on a drug's commercial success, they have every incentive to make their trials look as successful as possible because without the appropriate licence, companies are aware that years of research, time and massive amounts of money have to be thrown away and, in extremis, a company could even be financially broken by such failure. The sheer size of the gamble means that professional business ethics are bound to fly out of the window (266). In Colemans's opinion the pharmaceutical industry is "the most ruthless, most blatantly dishonest and most manipulative industry anywhere in the world. It makes the arms industry look positively angelic by comparison." (255)

Once a drug is approved for sale it becomes like any other product, whether one thinks of a brand of washing powder or a tin of soup. In order to become a commercial success, it obviously needs a maximum of advertising hype. Even though the industry likes us to believe that it spends most of its income on research for new medications, in reality, far more is spent on advertising and promoting already existing products. Even the industry's own executives admit that the success of the industry depends far more on creative marketing than on innovative research. Also, just as with any other commercial product, we will only learn its effectiveness, or its dangers, when it has been in general use for some time. And, as far as our medicines are concerned, it can take literally decades before a clear link can be established between a drug and consequent ill-effects.

The most worrying aspect of this pharmaceutical racket is that if anybody gets harmed by their medications, the industry is able to comfort themselves with the sure knowledge that even if they are sued, they are unlikely to lose. If all else fails, the industry will argue that, since the drug was granted a licence, the company cannot be held responsible because it did everyting it was expected to do by the relevant authorties (including animal experiments) when testing the safety of their products. The company can hardly be blamed, goes the argument, for any serious, or even lethal side-effects which only became apparent after the licence was granted (255).

Many may not even be aware that there is no law which states that drug manufacturers must use live animals to test the safety of their products. This is entirely their own choice because the industry has found that animal experiments are by far the quickest, cheapest, and easiest method to provide proof for the drug licencing authority that their product is 'non-toxic'. If we really wish to put a stop to these highly misleading and unscientific animal experiments, it is for us to demand that governments will declare animal experiments illegal!

This is certainly not going to be easy because the drug industry, by contributing a massive amount of capital to the treasure, is inexorably bound to the Western economies. It is therefore obvious that the last thing governments are prepared to do is upset the proverbial goose that lays all these golden eggs. Yet another factor that makes the abolition of vivisection not easy is because the pharmaceutical industry has been absolutely brilliant in promoting its usefulness. By using highly emotional blackmail such as 'would you rather save the life of your child or the life of a laboratory animal?', they have managed to convince almost everybody that without live animal experiments the human race will soon sink into oblivion.

A reason why the British government is particularly reluctant to get involved is because the Department of Health (DoH) maintains presently a highly conflicting role. On one hand, it is obliged to promote the pharmaceutical industry so that it will remain a profitable section of British commerce and, on the other, its role is to regulate the drug licencing prodecure so that dangerous and ineffective medications are not harming patients or wasting the scant resources of the National Health Service (NHS). Everyone can see that it is quite impossible to satisfy the pharmaceutical industry's demands for profits whilst safequarding the patients interests. This highly conflicting union is also the reason why governments are not prepared to take sides when consumers get harmed by prescribed medications (266).

However, the ever increasing NHS drug expenditure forced the government finally to introduce a so called 'limited list' of prescribable medications which consists only of the very basic ones, disregarding the more expensive modified versions collectively known as 'me-toos'. Considering that we have today, at any one time, up to 30,000 drugs on the market of which most are nearly identical apart from their brand names, at least that decision made sense. However, according to the World Health Organisation (WHO), only about 200 drugs are considered as being of some importance of which the United Nations Industrial Development Organisation lists only 26 as having a special priority (255). Admittedly the drug industry comes up sometimes with new products which, more often than not, are far too expensive to be purchased by our impoverished NHS (275).

There is no doubt that the National Health Service, when first introduced after the Second World War, was a wonderful concept. The basic thought behind it was that allowing the whole population free access to health care will lead to a healthier nation. However, something must have gone wrong somewhere because according to a fairly recent health analysis among nations, largely due to high death rates from cancer and heart disease, Britain is the unhealthiest nation among Western Europe and has also fallen behind Mexico and Taiwan (276).

It looks as if our National Health Service (NHS) has failed us on a colossal scale. Not only because it is already outsripping the country's ability to pay for it but also because it is making us more ill than ever before. As things are, our National Health Service (NHS) ought to be re-named as National Sickness Service which is far more appropriate. We are also in need of a National Health Service in its true sense of the word which unfortunately is not yet available. In the mean while, we can always improve our health by eating a nutritious whole-food diet and by avoiding toxic pollutants including synthetic medications.

CHAPTER 7

THE ILLNESS INDUSTRY

Before the existence of the modern medical establisment as we know it, practising clinicians fell into three basic categories. First, there were university-trained physicians who had acquired qualifications on the basis of their book work. The second group were surgeons who were allowed to do practically anything with a knife. The third group were apothecaries who were experts in preparing medications and who eventually became the first general practitioners (255).

Whilst applying their trade, these early doctors also invented and prepared their own medicaments, disregarding those which they found either harmful or ineffective. By continually searching for new compounds, it could be said that the work of these general practitioners was based on true scientific principles. This ideal situation began to change from 1844 when William Brockeden patented his pill- making machine which gave the doctors an opportunity to hand over their medicine preparations to the newly developing pill manufacturing industry. Though at the time they had a chance to retain control of the burgeoning drug industry, they chose not to get involved and the rest is history (255).

The main role of a modern doctor is to give a diagnosis and offer an appropriate treatment. In today's medical practice this is performed almost in a conveyer belt fashion where a diagnosis is almost invariably followed by a prescription. In fact, it has been estimated that 75% of doctors' consultations end up with one prescription drug or another even though up to 90% of people who visit their GPs are suffering from a so-called 'self-limiting' disorder which means that they will get well whether they have seen a doctor or not (256). So why are we receiving so many medications?

There is no question at all that the ultimate responsibilty relies on the pharmaceutical industry because it has managed to infiltrate its power to all corners of modern medicine. For example, it provides free information and education materials for medical schools. It supports scientific meetings and supplies free medicines and equipment to hospitals and surgeries. It finances, mainly through advertising, the publication of most medical journals. It spends colossal amounts of money on drug representatives which are known to lavish the medical profession with all kinds of free gifts from memo pads to expensive overseas functions. Also, most academic establishments, postgraduate centres and teaching hospitals are unable to continue their work without the sponsorship of the industry. Similarly universities and even whole departments within the NHS are equally indebted (266).

In addition, most modern medical research is either organised, paid for, commissioned, or subsidised by the industry. The pharmaceutical industry's financial take-over of medical research has had a particular sinister consequence because, being the major source of funds, it has the power to manipulate the direction of research in a way that shows that drugs are the only commodity in treating anything that is 'treatable' (266).

There is no doubt that the majority of doctors are sincere and caring people so they believe that the drugs they are prescribing are safe which, as we have seen, is not always the case. And, if something goes wrong, it seems to be the well-intending doctor who, due to 'prescribing error' or similar, is considered at fault if patients get harmed by medications, even though it is mostly us, the patients, who are really to blame for this colossal overprescribing. It has been estimated that seven out of ten prescriptions are written by doctors only because we hate to leave the surgery 'empty-handed' (277). In fact, most patients feel almost insulted if a doctor refuses to give them a prescription after consultation. For whatever reason, patients seem to imagine that doctors are not taking their ailments 'seriously' unless they are clutching that magic piece of paper after leaving the surgery. To these, who incidently account for the majority, the prescription is considered as a form of 'passport' to health. This is also why many doctors are almost obliged to invent 'an illness' and to prescribe something even though they are fully aware it is quite unnecessary.

The British National Formulary, published jointly by The British Medical Association and the Pharmaceutical Society, lists about 4,000 prescription drugs (151). As there are so many drugs available it is understandable that even the most caring and conscientious doctor cannot possibly have a good working knowledge of all of them. Considering that all synthetic medications are potentially toxic, it would require a special training to use them rationally and effectively. However, from the the earliest days at medical school, doctors' training concentrates mainly on the recognition of a disease whereas they learn hardly anything about clinical pharmacology. In fact, it is estimated that during the 5- year medical training, students receive only between one to twelve hours tuition on the subject of toxicology which is defined as 'the study of the harmful effects on man of exposure to chemicals as medicines, at work, at home, in food, and in the environment' (214). Nobody can expect that these few hours is sufficient to give doctors enough quidance on how to use medical drugs effectively, let alone to teach them how other toxic compounds such as pesticide residues, synthetic food additives, air pollution and heavy metal contamination can be responsible for so many health problems.

In the eyes of many patients a doctor is almost a god-like figure without whom the human race would soon sink into oblivion. This, almost holy alliance between doctor and patient, must also be the reason why many patients seem to get better even though a doctor has not prescribed him anything more potent than a simple sugar pill. This is known in medicine as the placebo effect (from Latin word 'please') which is based on a notion that hope and positive attitude have curative powers whereas worry and hopelessness do the opposite. Considering the blatantly treacherous nostrums early physicians used as 'medicines' such as animal dung, lizards's blood, powdered mummies etc, the history of medicine seems to contain not much else than this powerful healing effect of placebo.

In modern medicine this placebo effect is also known as psycho-neuro-immunology (PNI). Though both rest on the same idea that positive feelings make us healthy whereas negative ones cause ill health, there is neverthless a subtle difference. Unlike the placebo effect which is considered as being psychological, the healing effect of the PNI is based on findings that, through a complex biochemical and interactive energy-based network between the central nervous system and the immune system, thoughts are able to regulate how our immune system functions and hence, how our body deals with a disease (278, 279).

Besides synthetic medications, also other modern medical interventions can do us more harm than good. I have collected most information concerning dangers associated with vaccinations, x-rays, mammograms, cervical screening, blood transfusions, amniocentesis, chorionic villus sampling (CVS) and ultrasound monitoring from a book by Lynne McTaggart entitled "What Doctors Don't Tell You: The truth about the dangers of modern medicine" (280). Highly recommended!

Vaccinations:

The vaccination prodecure is seen by the medical profession as one of the greatest medical triumphs. Not only are we vaccinated against a whole host of diseases but these jabs are considered particularly vital for protecting babies against different kinds of childhood infections. In fact, under the present system there is tremendous pressure on parents to have their children vaccinated whether they like it or not. Doctors are even offered cash incentives the more children they are able to catch and vaccinate. However, just as there is no such as thing as a safe drug, there is no such a thing a safe vaccine. As vaccines represent the very epitome of modern medicine, most findings that dare to question the safety and validity of the prodecure are either suppressed or conveniently ignored. Besides Lynne McTaggart's book which is based on over 900 medical references, I have collected the following information from another well-referenced book by Leon Chaitow entitled "Vaccination and Immunisation: Dangers, Delusions and Alternatives" (281). Also highly recommended!

The dangers are **mumps** have been far exaggerated since the possibility of the accompanying symptoms of orchitis (inflamed testes) is almost neglible. Even if it occurs, it affects usually only one testis thereby leaving fertility intact. According to the German medical authorities, the mumps vaccine has been found to be responsible for 27 different neurological reactions including febrile seizures, unilateral deafness and encephalitis (280). In addition, reports in the US suggest that one out of every 100,000 children receiving mumps vaccination will develop meningitis as a direct result and a study from Yugoslavia puts the figure at one in every 1000 (280, 281).

German measles is not serious to children. It can however, be dangerous for an unborn child should a woman become infected during the early stages of pregnancy as it can lead the child being born with birth defects. However, studies have found that vaccinating young girls against German measles makes them more likely to contract the disease when they mature, because the vaccination prodecure seems to offer only partial protection, unlike the full protection they would have acquired if they were infected with the natural disease when young. As far as the vaccine itself is concerned, the medical profession has accepted, already for years, that it can lead to mild or, even crippling arthritic pains persisting for months and, in some instances, years (280, 281).

By the time immunisation was introduced on a mass scale in the mid-1950s against **whooping cough** (petrussis), mortality rates from this disease had already dropped by more than 80%. The same with other serious infections which began to decline well before vaccines were even invented (255, 280, 281). Of all vaccines, the petrussis/whooping cough vaccine is considered the most dangerous because it can lead to an irreversible brain damage. If the vaccine could really offer full protection against whooping cough the benefits might overweigh the risks but unfortunmately this is not the case (280, 281). For example, when a study examined the incidence of whooping cough cases in Canada and the United States, it found that nearly a half of the children who caught the disease had been fully vaccinated (280).

The same with **diptheria** vaccine. Instead of reducing infections, they seem to achieve just the opposite. For example, following the introduction of immunization against diptheria in Germany, diptheria cases soared from 40,000 to 250,000 per year and these were found mostly among vaccinated individuals (280). The **measles** vaccine seems to be equally useless. For example, during the 1985-86 measles outbreak in Britain, 60% of the cases were found among children who had been fully vaccinated (280).

One of the most worrying aspects of vaccination, particularly with the combined MMR (measles, mumps, rubella) vaccine, is that it has been associated with the development of autism (282). However, this was later discredited by a government-backed survey. Even though this was the case, parents' groups campaigning for research into possible dangers of the MMR vaccine were not reassured. They based their argument on that, during a ten year period, only 20 cases of autism were reported among children who had had the single measles vaccination. However, since the introduction of the MMR vaccine, the number of reported cases had soared to 1,800 (283).

Vaccination and SIDS:

Maybe the most frightening aspect of the vaccination prodecures is that it has also been linked with a Sudden Infant Death Syndrome (SIDS) (284). For example, when Dr William Torch, of the Unversity of Nevada School of Medicine, studied records of 103 infants who had died from SIDS, he noted that two thirds had received the DPT (diptheria, petrussis, tetanus) vaccine within the previous three weeks, many dying within a day. In his opinion this cannot be a coincidence but, at least in some cases, there must have been a causal relationship

(280, 281, 285). Yet another study undertaken in 1979 at the University of California Los Angeles (UCLA) under the sponsorship of the Food and Drug Administration, and subsequently confirmed by other studies, suggests that approximately 10-15% of the total number of SIDS deaths occurring annually in the USA could be attributed to the DPT vaccine (280, 281).

The reason why vaccines are dangerous, particularly for tiny infants, is because they not only contain viral particles but also many synthetic chemicals including neutralises, adjuvants and preservatives. Injecting this toxic concoction into a tiny baby whose body, brain and immune system are still at the very earliest stages of development, is bound to do him harm. Considering that most vaccinations are aimed at our defenceless infants, we ought to know precisely what we are doing!

In other words, according to Lynne McTaggart: "What the medical profession fails to tell you - Most doctors fervently believe that vaccines are one of the medical science's greatest success stories, responsible for wiping out many deadly infectious diseases of the past century. So steadfast is this faith that it prevents doctors from acknowledging evidence demonstrating ineffectiveness, adverse reactions and cases of a disease in children who have been vaccinated against it. In the 1994 UK campaign to inoculate all British children from five to 16 with measles, mumps and rubella jab, the Department of Health assured parents that side-effects to booster jabs were unlikely after being 'carefully studied by looking a large numbers of children in the United States'. In fact, the evidence on which this claim was based was rather more meagre. Before the campaign the DoH received a fax from officials at the US National Immunisation Programme explaining that the only evidence that boosters were safe was based on questionnaires sent to college students receiving boosters. What is worse, the UK's Public Health Laboratory Service completed a study before the campaign began, demonstrating that children given the measles, mumps and rubella jab were three times more likely to suffer from convulsions than those who didn't receive it. Two thirds of the cases of seizures were due to the measles component alone. Its findings were supported by a similar study carried out in America by the Centres of Disease Control (CDC) at about the same time. The CDC monitored the progress of 500,000 children across America, tapping into computerised records to discover adverse reactions to the two triple vaccines, the MMR and DPT (diphteria, petrussis, tetanus). It identified 34 major side-effects to the jabs, ranging from asthma, blood disorders, infectious diseases, diabetes and neurological disorders, including meningitis, polio and hearing loss. But it was the incidence of seizures that leapt off the graph. The rate increased three times above the norm within the first day of a child receiving the DDT shot, and rose 2.7 times within four to seven days of a child being given the MMR shot, increasing to 3.3 times within eight to 14 days."

"The success of vaccination is based entirely on assumption. Improved sanitation and hygiene, housing, better nutrition and isolation prodecures have occurred at the same time that vaccines have been introduced. The US Government notes that during the plague years of polio, 20,000 to 30,000 cases a year occurred in America, compared with 20 to 30 cases a year today. Neverthless, Dr Bernard Greenberg, head of the department of biostatics of the University of North Carolina School of Public Health, has said that polio increased by 50 per cent between 1957 and 1958 and 80 per cent from 1958 to 1959, after the introduction of mass immunisation. Despite the fact that the UK has had the MMR vaccine in place since 1988, and enjoys a high coverage among toddles, cases of measles recently were going up nearly one fourth. The zeal behind the measles campaign was founded on the belief that measles can be a life-threating condition. In America in 1990, at the height of the measles epidemic when 27,000 cases were reported, 89 died. But many deaths occurred among children of low-income families where poor nutrition played a part, as did failure to treat complications. In Africa, where children are markedly vitamin A deficient, measles does kill. However, as study after study demonstrates, even Third World children with adequate stores of vitamin A or those given vitamin A supplementation are likely to survive." (286).

Before this vaccination mania took hold, childhood infections were

126

considered to be a natural occurrence during every child's growth and development. In normally healthy children these infections just came and went leaving no after-effects except life-long immunity. So why suddenly this high-tech medical meddling? Let's face it, by far the best method for protecting children against infections of any kind is to breast-feed them for the first months of life to enhance their natural immunity. And therafter, to give them foods that contain all the necessary vitamins, minerals and essential fatty acids needed for an effective immune system function. Besides sound nutrition, Leon Chaitow lists in his book other alternatives that are known to potentiate immunity including homeopathic and herbal remedies (281).

And last but not least, it must be stressed that neither Lynne McTaggart, Leon Chaitow nor I are offering advice either for or against immunisation. The only point we are trying to make is that the validity of the vaccination prodecure should be questioned in more detail and before any further conclusions can be drawn, everyone ought to receive a clear and definite answer at least to the following questions. First of all, are vaccinations well and truly safe? Secondly, do they really offer protection against the diseases they are given for?

X-rays:

All radiation is harmful and x-rays are no exception. Even so, x-rays are taken almost routinely though it has been estimated that at least 20% of the examinations are clinically useless in the sense that the results give no medically useful information (280). The main problem with this prodecure is that the body will never 'forget' its radiation dose and so the harm is cumulative. In other words, the more x-rays are taken, the more serious is the damage. Considering that radiation is linked with the formation of cancers, we ought to make sure that we are not exposed to it more often than absolutely necessary. The unborn child is particularly vulnerable, therefore x-rays are never given to women whilst pregnant because it can lead to the baby being born malformed and/or mentally retarded (280).

Mammograms:

Another x-ray prodecure is the mammography which is used to screen early malignancies in the breast tissue. Though well intended, some research evidence shows that mammograms may do more harm than good as they can cause the very disease they are intended to detect. In fact, some studies have found a higher death rate from breast cancers in the mammogram screened group compared to those who detected their cancer through self-examination. This is thought to come about because radiation may be responsible for spreading the malignant cancer cells faster, thereby hastening the disease process (280).

Another problem linked with mammogram examinations is a high rate of inaccuracy because, just as with other x-rays, the results depend entirely on who is doing the reading. It is not suprising therefore that sometimes malignant lumps are missed, and other times they are 'detected' even though they are not present (280). Considering that the test results are unreliable it is vital that every woman who participates in this screening programme should neverthless continue regular self-examininations for any breast abnormalities.

This high level of inaccuracy may also be a reason why mammography has not made a great deal of difference to the actual breast cancer survival rates. In fact, breast cancer mortality has remained more or less unchanged despite these costly and well-intended efforts to improve early detection and consequent treatment (280). Some even suggest that regular screening for breast cancer ought to be discontinued because the number of lives saved is too tiny to justify the unnecessary worry and anxiety which millions of women go through because their mammograms are found to be slightly 'suspicious'. In fact, it is estimated that about one in 20 mammograms show signs of 'malingancies' which, after a further examination, 80-93 per cent turn out to be false alarms (287).

Cervical screening:

As with mammography, cervical screening has been touted as being the only reason why deaths from this cancer have declined. However, this assumption seems to be incorrect because not only did the incidence of cervical cancers begin to decline before the mass screening programme was introduced but also because since the screening began, the death rates from this type of cancer have remained stubbornly at about 2,000 cases per year. As with mammography, the reason is thought to be a high level of inaccuracy as there seems to be an equal chance that abnormal cells are missed or that normal cells are detected as 'cancerous' which are not (280).

Regardless that the number of women screened for cervical cancer has risen from 22 per cent in 1988 to 93 per cent in 1993, this has done no difference to cervical cancer death rates. Some experts are already questioning whether cervical screening ought to be discontinued because, as with mammography, the inaccuracy of the prodecure and the number of false-positives, create a great deal of unnecessary worry and anxiety among millions of women. It is estimated that of approximately 5 million smears performed in Britain each year, about 7 per cent are found to be 'abnormal' to some degree (288).

Besides a possible error in detection, there is also a great deal of controversy as to what to do if pre-cancerous cells are detected. Depending on the school of thought, some doctors advocate immediate treatment whereas others prefer to keep on monitoring the situation to see whether the cells will revert back to normal, which is often the case. In fact, it is estimated that about 50 per cent of the women from whom a minor abnormality has been detected during the first test, will subsequently have a normal one the next time around. One reason for these transient abnormalities could be a low-level infection which resort back to normal as the soon the inflammation subsides (289).

Blood transfusions:
Though blood transfusion have been practised for centuries, it has never been subjected to proper double-blind scientific experiments to find out whether it has any benefits (280). The most common 'transfusion trigger' is a low haemoglobin level even though studies have found that most patients are able to tolerate intermittently low haemoglobin providing that the circulating blood volume is kept up with artificial fluid-

volume expanders. In fact, it has been estimated that most adults can lose up to a third of their total blood volume and not go into irreversible shock providing that the haemodilution is kept constant (280). The main problem associated with blood transfusions is the danger of contracting different types of blood-borne infections from contaminated blood products. Considering that blood is such an individual commodity it is always best to recieve one's own. Therefore, anyone waiting for surgery ought to donate his own blood ahead of the time (290).

Now just a few words of prenatal tests such as amniocentesis, chorionic villus sampling (CVS) and ultrasound monitoring which have been designed to detect whether a foetus carries chromosomal abnormalities or is otherwise malformed.

Amniocentesis:

Amniocentesis involves having a needle inserted into the abdomen to draw out amniotic fluid which is then tested in the laboratory for possible chromosomal abnormalities. A drawback of this test is a long waiting period because is not usually performed until the sixteenth week of pregnancy. It then takes another two to three weeks before the final results are available. This means that if abnormalities are found to be present and the woman prefers not to continue with the pregnancy, this would entail a second-trimerster abortion with the maximum of physical and psychological ramifications. Another concern with this test is that it is associated with an increased rate of miscarriages. In fact, it has been estimated that the miscarriage risk may be as high as one in a hundred (280).

Chorionic villus sampling (CVS):

When chorionic villus sampling (CVS) became available it was thought to be an answer to every mother-to-be's prayer as it can be performed between the ninth and twelfth week of pregnancy. However, a problem with this test is that it has been associated with a relatively high incidence of limb malformations (280).

Ultrasound monitoring:
Ultrasound was first developed during the second World War to track down enemy submarines. Today, it is used to track down babies in the womb when they are only at the tadpole stage. Although originally designed to monitor high-risk pregnancies, today it is used like a TV-set where the unborn foetus plays the leading role. Although there is no clear evidence that the prodecure represents a risk to the unborn child, neither is there a quarantee that it is perfectly safe. At least, studies 'in vitro' have shown that ultrasound is able to damage the cell structure as well as produce changes in the cellular DNA. Furthermore, when pregnant animals have been exposed to ultrasound, it led to the pups being born with a lowered birth weight and delayed muscular development. Whether this only happens with animal babies, only time will tell. Until then, according to Lynne McTaggart, every would-be-mother ought be aware that by exposing her unborn child to ultrasound she is participating in one of the biggest laboratory experiments in modern medical history (280). Considering that literally thousands of babies are born every day all over the world without being monitored, pricked, peered and hazzled whilst developing in the comfort of their mothers' wombs, why suddenly all this fuss? Better leave them alone just as nature intended!

Hospitals:
Even hospitals can be dangerous for our health. For example, a study conducted at 19 large hospitals in England and Wales found that, due to lax hygiene standards, 60,000 non-surgical patients a year catch serious infections in hospital, with mothers in maternity wards and patients in intensive care units most at risk (291). Another survey found that hospital infections are responsible for at least 5,000 deaths a year and partly responsible for a further 15,000. Also that, on average, one patient in sixteen becomes infected (292). Not only that but others have found that hospital food is so low in nutritional value that it leads to malnutrition which in turn does not only prolong the healing process but can be responsible for the development of secondary illnesses, even

death (283). It looks that hospitals can be pretty dangerous places even for perfectly healthy individuals let alone for those who are not feeling well at all. As things are, one would have thought that hospitals are the very last place a sick person should go looking for 'treatment'.

The gene theory:
Just a few words about 'gene-theory' which is hailed nowadays as the greatest triumph in modern medical history. Hardly a day goes by without scientists discovering one gene or another. By following the press headlines only, this newly- found theory gives an impression that the human race is nothing but a bunch of genes with minds of their own. It does not matter how healthy or happy we are, it seems that our genes always have the last word. For example, "Scientists identify gene linked with depression", "Cause of wet beds traced to gene", "Scientists find kidney disease gene", "Alzheimer's gene is identified", "Scientists identify breast cancer genes", "Secret happiness may be in genes", "Slimmers told to abandon guilt and blame the genes", "Bad- tempered and extravagant? Blame it on genes", "Don't fret about worry, it is all in your genes" and so on and so forth.

This ever increasing ability to identify all types of genes might be commendable from the scientific point of view but what is it supposed to achieve as far we ordinary mortals are concerned? By blaming our genes for bad temper, a feeling of happiness or extravagancy makes no sense at all. Blaming them for the development of Alzheimer's disease or cancer is downright depressing. Not only because waiting for these illnesses to appear will cause tremendeous worry and anxiety but also because, at least to date, there are no effective treatments.

However, it looks as if these 'gene-scares' which so far have managed to frighten thousands of people out of their minds, have hardly any foundation at all because the development of most disease processes never relies on one gene alone but always involves a complicated interaction of 10, 100, 1,000 or more genes at one time (294). Even in cases where a genetic connection can be traced, researches have found that genes never act in isolation but always in connection with the environment (294-296).

Also, according to Professor Emeritus Thoday, any diseases that is claimed to be caused by a single defect in the genetic code is relatively rare. Another flaw in this gene- theory is that a disease can be caused by different genes in different families. Not only that, but taking Alzheimer's disease, for example, which so far has been associated with three different genes, offers only the opportunity of identifying three different components of the underlying biochemistry of the disease. Therefore, what hope is there of understanding the more common diseases whose causation is not only caused by numbers of genes but environmental factors as well? (297)

It is estimated that the human genome (formed from words gene and chromosome) contains approximately 100,000 genes which are wrapped around 23 pairs of chromosomes that are made of about 3 billion pairs of DNA which themselves are composed of four chemical molecules (bases): adenine, thymine, cytosine and guanine. The Human Genome Project (HGP) is designed to localize the 100,000 genes within the genome as well as to determine the order of bases along the DNA strand. Considering that the human genome is made up of about three billion pairs of DNA which in turn are equipped with 'fixed points' such as telomeres and centromeres which stops the DNA 'fraying', it will take a hell of a long time before scientist are able to figure out what each bit is up to. Also that genes alone are not responsible for the development of complex disease processes such as cancers, Alzheimer's, heart disease and so forth, but environmental factors play an equal part, the time needed to figure out subsequent gene- environmental interactions will surely take another eternity. In other words, considering the incomprehensive complexity involved in the causation of most degenerative diseases, it is best to stop worrying, leave the scientists to it and eat drink and be merry!

CHAPTER 8
IS MEDICINE A SCIENCE?

I have mentioned that even though I suffered from the same group of symptoms for years, both diagnoses and treatments changed not only from one country to another but also from one doctor to the next. It was not until I came across a book by Lynn Payer entitled "Medicine & Culture: Notions of Health and Sickness" that I found an answer to this perplexing dilemma (298). The author is an American journalist with a background in biochemistry who had covered medical topics all over Europe, Canada and the United States.

Whilst working in Europe, not only did she notice striking differences between European and American medical practices but also considerable variations among the European medical profession which prompted her to conduct a thorough investigation to find out why medical practices between countries are so inconsistent. Her book covers French, German, British and the American medicine and culture (298). Highly recommended!

Our usual encounters with doctors are not prompted by rare diseases but with common everyday problems such as vague aches and pains, excessive fatigue, palpitations, dizziness, feelings of anxiety, depression and so on. In fact, many visit their GPs complaining of a similar cluster of symptoms to those I suffered for years. According to Lynn

Payer's book, if I had seen a doctor in France the diagnosis would most likely have been spasmophilia, which is a French description for anxiety neurosis and which is usually treated with magnesium supplements. This may be just a coincidence but a condition known as chronic fatigue syndrome (CFS) is also thought to be associated with low blood magnesium levels (299).

If I had consulted a doctor in Germany, I would have probably been diagnosed as suffering from vasovegative dystonia which is used as a 'polite diagnosis' for patients who complain of multiple symptoms without outward clinical signs and who otherwise might receive a diagnosis of psychiatric disorder of some kind. In fact, the German medical profession is very much opposed to diagnose anyone as mentally ill, preferring, whenever possible, to describe a mental disorder in physical terms (298). This German reluctance to use psychiatric diagnoses seems to be also the reason why less than 1% of German patients are considered as having mental health problems as opposed to Britain where nearly a quarter of the population are considered mentally ill (71).

Another widely used diagnosis in Germany is low blood pressure (hypotension), also known as myocardial insufficiency. Neither the British nor the American medical profession recognise low blood pressure as a disease. Just the very opposite. Anyone who has low blood pressure either in Britain or in America is considered exeptionally healthy. However the German medical profession takes even marginally low blood pressure seriously. So much so that they have over eighty different medications to treat the condition most of which contain adrenaline (298).

I found this particularly interesting because reactive hypoglycaemia (low blood sugar) is also associated with low blood pressure. Likewise, it is known to lead to a mild form of adrenal insufficiency. Considering that most medicines used in Germany for treating low blood pressure contain adrenaline which has the ability to raise both blood pressure and blood sugar levels, it is not inconceivable that this German 'myocardial insufficiency' is only a sign of underlying reactive hypoglycaemia which, as we already know, can be treated simply and effectively by dietary means (77-79, 84).

If I had consulted a doctor in the United States the diagnosis would most likely have been neurasthenia which is considered as a true 'American disease' (298). However, neurasthenia is also known in medical literature by other names including anxiety neurosis, hyperventilation syndrome, phobic-anxiety depersonalization syndrome, neurocirculatory asthenia, effort syndrome, cardiac neurosis, irritable heart, nervous exhaustion and DaCosta's syndrome (84). Furthermore, it is interesting to note that the symptoms of neurasthenia, also known as anxiety neurosis, hyperventilation syndrome and so on and so forth are more or less the same as those associated with chronic fatigue syndrome (CFS), food/chemical allergies and reactive hypoglycaemia (84).

However, the American medical profession treats their neurasthenia, and anything else that is treatable, with great gusto. They do more diagnostic tests and perform more operations than anywhere else in the world. Every disease in America must be conquered, if not by operating something out then by putting plenty of medicines in. Not only do they have to do something but they also have to do it fast! A true victim of the American 'can-do-and-must-do' approach is a passive patient who refuses to get sucked into this mad medical-merry-go-round. One observer remarked that a calm and placid patient is really in trouble because rush and desperate cheerfulness are the only acceptable signs which prove that the patient is trying to do at least something positive to improve his health. The American medical profession has also declared chemical warfare against 'mental illnesses' resulting in more psychotropic drugs being prescribed in that country than anywhere else in the world (298).

One of the most fascinating aspects of medicine is how different cultures perceive the same behaviour patterns. For example, when a study compared opinions of French and British psychiatrists of the same group of symptoms it was amazing how cultural differences alone influence the diagnostic outcome. When the French studied the list of symptoms they picked only those as 'treatable' which showed passive emotions such as lack of energy, loss of interest and difficulties in making decisions. The British psychiatrists accepted passive feelings readily but declared all symptoms as 'treatable' which indicated an excitable behaviour pattern such as agitation, irritability, anger or excitability (298).

This may also be the reason why people of foreign extraction are often diagnosed as 'mentally ill' in Britain. According to one press report, it is estimated that at least one in ten patients in London suffering from mental health problems are foreigners. Not only that they add to the capital's shortage of hospital beds but, when discharged, they are left to roam the streets increasing the risk to the British public (300). It is also believed that immigrants and their children with Afro-Caribbean backgrounds are five times more likely to develop schizophrenia compared to other population groups (301). Though this kind of cultural segregation is still rife in Britain, the American Psychiatric Association (APA) has notified its members that people from different cultural backgrounds have different mental problems. In their new set of guidelines, APA has stated that mental-health profession should always take into consideration both cultural and ethnic origins of their patients before a diagnosis is made (302). Let's hope that the British psychiatric profession will follow suit before all our mental health wards become over-saturated with excitable foreigners.

Not only are mental health problems perceived differently from one country to another, the same applies with some major illnesses. For example, a study by the World Health Organisation (WHO) found that doctors from different countries gave different explanations when shown identical information from the same death certificates. In most instances they tended to disagree except in cases of cancer though the location of the cancer was sometimes disputed. In other words, as one observer remarked: "Plenty of people are still dying of diseases which other people don't even believe in." (298).

So how can medicine, which is considered as a form of science, vary so much from one country to another? The answer is that while medicine does benefit from scientific input, cultural aspects of any given country seem to intervene at every step of the way. The other question that comes to mind is that even though the culture of medicine can differ so much between countries why don't they intermix more readily with the relative ease of modern communication technology? The answer seems to be that even though the technology is available and doctors are indeed aware of what is going on elsewehere, the news is neverthless often ignored because every country's medical profession far prefers to 'discover' something themselves than to take notice of other countries' medical findings (298).

This attitude of rather not knowing what others have been up to has obviously resulted in countries continuously 'discovering' aspects of medical research which another country has known for years. Also, because competition is rife, if a country has found something ahead of another, this is usually met with a rather high-handed and dismissive attitude. For example, when an American doctor was questioned about a new treatment regime discovered in Europe, his reply was: "Our first reaction is bound to be negative. We are very chauvinistic and have the attitude that if we haven't discovered something, it is probably wrong" (298).

For the same reason the medical profession is generally not that interested in reading other countries' medical literature. When British, French and German doctors were interviewed about their reading habits no British doctor could name even one French or German medical journal whereas the French and the Germans could name 'The Lancet'. Not one French doctor knew the name of any German medical journal and vice versa which is really not that suprising due to the language barrier. The communication between the British and the American medical profession is better but even they seem to prefer to read their own. This became apparent when an American doctor was asked whether he was interested in reading British medical journals. His reply was: "We don't read much foreign medical literature here" (298).

There are also considerable differences between nations regarding clinical trials. The British medical profession prefers theory and data collecting above individual considerations. This respect for theory, coupled with a philosophy that society should take precedence over an individual, has led the British medical profession to become the chief proponents of the so-called randomised-double- blind-placebo-controlled-cross-over-trials-with-matched-controls. According to the French medical profession: "English doctors are the accountants of the medical world" (298).

However, if a study is aimed to be published in a British medical journal, doctors from other countries are aware that they also have to use these randomised-double-blind-cross-over-trials-with-matched-controls. Anyhow, whilst it is quite acceptable in Britain to divide a group of patients into a treatment and a placebo group, the American medical profession finds this unethical because it holds a view that only treatment is the name of the game. Instead of 'dummy pills', American medical trials prefer to compare different treatment methods against one another (298).

Another cultural difference between the British and the American medical profession is that once the trial has been completed, British doctors tend to draw far less sweeping conclusions from the results compared with their American counterparts. For example, when a study discussed a specific cholesterol-lowering drug, the British medical profession decided that the drug could only be prescribed for those who had similar cholesterol levels as in the original research whilst the American medical profession extrapolated that the drug is useful for anyone suffering from raised cholesterol, whatever the reading. The same with a blood pressure lowering drug. The British doctors concluded that the drug can only be used for treating men of a certain age, whereas the Americans decided that it is equally useful for treating everyone regardless of age, sex or blood pressure measurements (298).

The same happened with a large-scale trial which was testing whether Tamoxifen can either prevent or delay the development of breast cancer. The American researchers decided to abandon the trial fourteen months before the agreed date because they decided in their infinite wisdom that the Tamoxifen-treated group had lower breast cancer rates compared to the placebo group. Resulting that the British medical profession got pretty fed-up because, according to them, this premature publication from the United States is bound to put back any meaningful results of the trial, at best, by four years (303). And talking about 'meaningful results'. Tamoxifen does not only cause liver tumours in rats but it also greatly increases the development of cancer in the lining of the womb in the human species (274).

Some members of the medical profession claim that they are able to stay on top of other countries' medical advances by attending international conferences. However, these also can have their drawbacks. Not because of a language barrier as most gatherings use English, but largely because diagnostic terms can have so many different meanings. In France for example, patients never have headaches only migraines. In Germany nobody suffers from chest pains, only heart pains. Also, if a German doctor speaks about myocardiac insufficiency he is not even discussing the heart but that a patient has low blood pressure which, as far as the British and the American medical professions are concerned, is not even an illness but a sign of excellent health (298).

Similar discrepancies are found in psychiatric language. Take schizophrenia for example, which refers to widely varied concepts in different countries which has meant that the national incidence of this condition varies greatly from one country to the next. The same with drug addiction. Some countries consider drug addiction as a 'disease', some as a punishable criminal behaviour and others look at it as just a way of life (304).

Another notable cultural difference between French, German, British and American medicine is so called 'virus theory'. Neither the French nor the German medical profession are not that keen in viruses. They do not deny that viral infections can lead to ill-health, but only when the health of an individual is already compromised. This in turn has had the effect that they usually 'treat' viral infections by advising patients how best to strenghten their own immunity so that it can deal with the offending bugs effectively. This is usually achieved by prescribing different health-promoting tonics, homeopathy, herbal medicine, spa treatments and such like. In fact, it has been estimated that about 6,000 French doctors prescribe homeopathic medication of which about half are using homeopathic remedies exclusively. Likewise, about one-fifth of German doctors practice either homeopathy and/or herbal medicine. As the French and the German medical profession seem to be more interested in promoting health than by curing a disease, it is not suprising that their top-twenty prescription 'drugs' include several health promoting tonics, as opposed to the British and the American top-twenty which mentions none (298).

Unlike their French and German counterparts, both the British and the American medical profession are exceptionally keen on viruses. Doctors are fully aware that only bacterial, not viral infections, respond to antibiotic medication but as it is often impossible to determine at the onset of an illness whether it is bacterial or viral in origin, many doctors tend to give up in the face of the whining patient and prescribe antibiotics 'just in case'. This trend of prescribing antibiotics for the most trivial of complaints, has resulted in an ever increasing development of antibiotic-resistant bacteria, popularly known as 'superbugs' against which no antibiotic can prevail. According to a group of international scientists, the growing number of bacteria that cannot be treated with any antibiotic may soon be responsible for global health crisis. Already for millions of people standard antibiotic treatment is failing to work because new strains of bacteria have developed multidrug resistance. According to Julian Davies of the University of British Columbia, Vancouver: 'During the past 50 years we have been involved in an incredible experiment. Tens of billions of pounds of antibiotics have been released on this planet. The globe is bathed in a dilute solution of antibiotics. You might expect all microbes to have been killed. But they are not killed, they have become 'resistant'" (305).

This rapid emergence of bacterial resistance arises because antibiotics exert a selective pressure on bacteria by eliminating those which are sensitive and leaving behind an aberration which begins to multiply and to colonise the space left behind. The reason why some bacteria can survive is because antibiotics are designed to demolish their protective cell wall. However, to fight back, these insolent creatures have adopted a gamut of tricks. Not only have they managed to grow cell walls that are practically impenetrable but they also have learned to renew their wall-building proteins at such a fast rate that they are able to withstand and survive most antibiotic battering. Anyone interested in this fascinating subject ought to read Geoffrey Cannon's book "Superbug: Nature's Revenge" (306).

Some years ago when sauntering around a car-boot sale, I happened to come across a remarkable book by Harry Benjamin entitled "Everybody's Guide to Natural Cure" (307) which was first published in 1936 and re-printed several times until 1946. The author is a naturopath by profession who believes that the reason for most illnesses are: inadequate nutrition, environmental pollution, insufficient exercise, rest and relaxation. He writes: "One would imagine, from the way the medical profession speak, that one tiny little germ or bacillus (countless of thousands of which could scarely cover a head of a pin) has only to enter the body of a healthy individual, for that individual to be stricken with some fell disease or another. Perhaps typhoid! Perhaps cancer! And modern man goes around terrified out of his life because of the existance of these tiny creatures which he endows with such malevoent properties, and which he believes are always threatening him, and which only the most powerful microscope can reveal to his shuddering gaze. What nonsense it all is. Our bodies are always full of germs and bacteria; they play a most important part in the workings of the body, especially in the destructive processes. For constructive and destructive processes are always going on within the body, night and day, asleep or awake, whether we know it or not"

"When Pasteur elaborated his celebrated germ theory of disease, the whole medical world enthusiastically and unhesitatingly accepted it, in full belief that there at last was the conclusive solution to the vexed problem of disease, the solution they have long been waiting for. At last the dreaded disease was fully established. It was germs! Disease was due to germ infection. All one had to do was to kill the germs, and disease would disappear. But fifty years of adherence to the germ theory and despite literally astonishing feats of bacteriological science, disease exerts as firm hold upon humanity as heretofore. The germs appear to thrive better than their victims. Pasteur, because of the superficial plausibility of his germ theory, has set the whole medical fraternity on a wild-goose chase which is leading nearer and nearer to the brink of futility understanding and treatment of disease. Why? Because Medical science has always looked to externals for the cause of disease, instead of factors at work within the body of the individual concerned. Consequently, despite its skill and honesty of purpose, the medical profession continues to add error to error, and pile up enormity upon enormity, in attempting to 'cure' disease by means of administration of poisonous drugs and vaccines, and the very drastic employment of the surgeon's knife, without having the faintest idea that what it is inevitably doing is really adding to the disease bill of the nation, rather than substracting from it."

"One only has to pay a flying visit to any hospital or busy panel doctor's waiting room, or watch the stream of cars continually rolling up to various doctors in Harley Street, or read the patent medicine advertisements in the newspapers, to realise that the world's disease problem is still waiting to be solved at medical hands. Indeed, it appears to be growing more and more insoluble every day. Although called 'science', orthodox medicine has never been able to formulate any definite rules or principles governing the appearance of disease in the human body, or how it might overcome. It has always proceeded by the method known as 'trial and error', with disease exerting a wider and ever firmer grip all the time. What is considered 'fashionable' form of treatment in one decade is superseded the next by a different form, and the 'blood-letting and leaching' which were the chief theraupetic agencies in their time, are sneered at by a later generation of medicos who pin their faith to deadly dangerous drugs and the 'surgeon's knife'. On the surface these methods appear to be doing something, the cutting and slashing and dosing and doping appear to achieve results; so that even the medical profession is genuinely believing that it is actually overcoming disease, until the yearly statistics are looked at!"

143

"The mass and mankind has the most touching and implicit belief in the 'wonder-working' powers of 'the Doctor'. The word of the 'Great Medical Authority' is accepted without cavil or question by all matters relating disease. The medical profession is universally revered for its great and unselfish work of 'ridding' the world of suffering and ill-health, simply because the public knows nothing about what is really happening when it places itself so completely into medical hands. Besides, if medical theory and practice is known to be wrong, the world would feel itself utterly lost. For who else would there be to turn to help humanity in its continual struggles with disease, if one could no longer rely on the doctor? No one who has not tried can understand the almost utter hopelessnes of attempting to convey these simple truths to the conventionally-minded people of today, steeped as they are in implicit belief as to the wonder-working powers of 'the Doctor', accepting everything he says with childish faith and obedience, as coming from one who surely knows all there is to know about disease, its causes and cures, absolutely convinced as to the efficiency and healing value of the multi-colored medicines they trustingly carry home with them after visit to the surgery, speaking with bated breath of 'great specialists' and miraculous eleventh-hour operations performed at moment's notice which has saved lives of near and dear ones, fully satisfied that the ills they suffer from are nothing whatever to do with their habits of living or the food they eat, but are due to nasty pernicious germs, sent by perverse Providence to harass them. No one, I repeat, who has not tried can understand the hoplessness of trying to convince people such as these (and they make fully ninety-nine per cent of the population of all civilized countries) that medical practice - based, as it is, upon a completely erroneous philosophy of disease. Despite its skill, knowledge, position, prestige, power, authority and so called 'achievements' in alleviating the suffering of humanity, is really and truly a menace, and a most insidious menace, be noted, to the health and welfare of the society, by actually intensifying disease instead of overcoming it" (307).

The reason why I have quoted Harry Benjamin at length is because nothing has changed in sixty years since the book was written. The world's disease problems are still waiting to be solved in medical hands. Indeed, they appear to be growing more and more insoluble every day. Why? Because the medical science is still looking for externals for the cause of disease production instead of the factors at work within the body of the patient concerned. Even today, despite its skill and honesty of purpose, the medical profession continues to add error to error in attempting to 'cure' disease by prescribing poisonous drugs and vaccines, without having the faintest idea that what it is inevitably doing is really adding to the disease bill of the nation, rather than substracting from it.

Moreover, this decline will continue as long as we carry on treating our precious body as if it were some kind of banger vechicle which can be driven as recklessly and fast one pleases, and when troubles loom, expect a doctor to repair it, patch it up, or at worst, to sign a death certificate!

CHAPTER 9

THE FORESIGHT SOLUTION

Todays's health care profession seems to be concerned about reproduction from two completely opposing angles. They have either family planning services or antenatal services, the latter becoming interested in caring for the future mother and child after the baby has developed in the womb for some weeks which is already too late because the human foetus goes through its fastest growth-spurt between gestation and its very first four weeks of life. Already by the 26th day, the foetal arm buds have appeared followed by leg buds a couple of days later. In the third week, the tiny embryo has a spinal cord and a miniscule beating heart. At four weeks it has grown rudimentary eyes, ears, a mouth, and a brain and it also has simple kidneys, liver, digestive tract and a blood stream.

This means that having missed one or two periods, and by the time a wuman seeks maternity care services, most of her baby's vital organs have already been formed or malformed. Most of us already know that if the would-be mother is short of folic acid at the time when the foetal spinal cord is closing, which takes place at around the third week of pregnancy, this can result in the baby being born with spina bifida. However, folic acid is not the only vitamin needed to produce a healthy infant, others are equally important. The same with minerals. Not only maternal vitamin and mineral deficiencies can harm the unborn child but similarly environmental toxins have an ability to depress, slow down and/or disorganise the foetal cell replication processes which are resposible for most birth malformations.

The same nutritional principles applies to the future father because it takes about four months for the male sperm, which carries the genes, to grow into maturity. If the male is malnourished and/or his body harbours too many environmental toxins whilst his sperm commences this maturation process, the health of his sperm cannot be guaranteed. A toxic and malnourished sperm is either infertile or, if it achieves conception, the genes may be so badly damaged that the baby is born malformed.

Whenever would-be parents are asked whether they would prefer a boy or a girl, the answer is usually that they do not mind as long as the baby is born healthy. In those unfortunate situations where an infant is born malformed, this tragedy is considered as being 'a quirk of nature' against which we had no power to act. This is not true. Every animal breeder knows that the only way to secure the birth of a healthy offspring is to mate two healthy animals together. Yet, when this is mentioned to would-be human parents, all one tends to get back is a suprised stare!

The Foresight approach:
Foresight, the Association for the Promotion of Preconceptual Care, a registered charity, was formed in 1978 by Mrs Belinda Barnes. Its main objective is to promote preconception care advice designed to reduce and if possible, to eliminate, from both future parents all the potentially harmful influences that are known to compromise the baby's health from the earliest days of life. Their preconception care programme focuses primarily on the following areas: nutritional deficiencies, heavy metal toxicities, alcohol, cigarette smoking, synthetic food additives, pesticide pollution and genito-urinary infections. They also have other areas of concern such as food and/or chemical allergies, malapsorption syndrome, intestinal parasites, natural methods of contraception and so on. I am obviously unable to discuss here all aspects

regarding Foresight's work but will only mention the very basics. Anybody interested in studying the subject in detail ought to read the following books: "Planning for a Healthy Baby: Essential reading for all Future Parents" (308), "Preparation for Pregnancy: An Essential Guide" (309) and/or a booklet entitled "Health Professionals' Guide to Preconception Care" (310). The first book is written with the general public in mind whereas the second, as well as the booklet, are more suitable for health professionals.

Nutritional deficiences:

Thousands of animal experiments have shown that the most commonly seen birth defects, such as spina bifida, heart defects, cleft palate, club foot, etc., can be either re-produced, or eliminated, by diet alone (311). Just a few examples. It must be stressed, however, that animal experiments relating to human health can be misleading and results are only accurate regarding the species experimented on.

Water soluble vitamins:

Maternal folic acid deficiency is linked in animal studies with miscarriage, deformed limbs, hydrocephalus, anencephaly, spina bifida, cleft palate and harelip. Also with heart, skeletal, lung and brain malformations (311). In human babies maternal folic acid deficiency has been found to be resposible for spina bifida, hydrocephalus, anencephaly, cleft palate and harelip (308, 309). However, folic acid is not the only water-soluble vitamin required to produce a healthy infant. For example maternal vitamin B1 (thiamine) deficiency has been linked in animal studies with infertility, perinatal mortality and small birth weight offspring and vitamin B2 (riboflavin) deficiency is associated with sterility, stillbirths, blood disorders, kidney defects, cleft palate, small foetuses and both limb and skeletal malformations (311).

Fat soluble vitamins:

Maternal vitamin E deficiency in animal studies has been found to cause hydrocephalus and both limb and heart malformations. Also, if pregnant animals are kept on a low vitamin A diet, the pups are born with hydrocephalus and a variety of eye, heart and genital abnormalities (311). Even though animal studies have shown how dangerous maternal vitamin A deficiency can be for the developing offspring, pregnant women are warned against eating vitamin A-rich foods because they are also associated with birth malformations. Indeed, an excessive vitamin A intake is harmful for the unborn child but so is a deficiency. In short, as in everything regarding nutrition, moderation is always the key.

Zinc:

All essential mineral deficiencies are also linked, both in animal experiments and human studies, with reproductive failures (308, 309). For example, maternal zinc deficiency has been found to be responsible for a wide variety of birth malformations encompassing every organ system in the body. This is not suprising because zinc is centrally involved in most events relating to cell division and replication (114, 115). For example, animal experiments have shown that maternal zinc deficiency can lead the pups being born with malformations affecting most internal organs including brain, heart and lungs (114, 115).

In humans, ever increasing research evidence has linked maternal zinc deficiency with prematurity and a low birth weight (115, 308, 309, 312). This was proven again by an American research experiment which measured the effect of zinc supplements on the birth weight of 580 babies. About half of the women were given every day dietary supplements without zinc whereas the others, randomly selected, received supplements which also contained 25mg of zinc. The results show that the babies born to women taking the zinc were significantly heavier at birth compared to the babies born to mothers not receiving zinc. Some of the improvement in the birth weights of babies born to mothers taking zinc was associated with a lower rate of premature deliveries. But even when allowance was made for the prematurity, mothers taking zinc had larger babies compared with the non- supplemented group (313). Not only that maternal zinc deficiency is associated with low birth weight and premature delivery, it is also known to lead to a reduced immune system function in the newborn. In males, low zinc status can be responsible for a low sperm count and infertility (115, 308, 309).

Iron:
Just a few words about low maternal iron levels which are also associated with reproductive failures. As a precaution, if the maternal haemoglobin level is found to be below 10g/dl, she is usually prescribed iron supplements. However, some research evidence suggests that this practice may do more harm than good. For example, when a study analysed in restrospect 150,000 pregnancies regarding maternal haemoglobin levels and compared them to infant prematurity and birth weight, it found that a haemoglobin level of about 9.5g/dl seems to be associated with an optimum health of an infant. More suprisingly, the study found that a failure of the maternal haemoglobin level to fall below 10.5g/dl indicated a greater risk of a low birth weight and/or premature delivery (314). The reason for this strange phenomenon is not clear but it has been suggested that the low maternal haemoglobin level reflects an increased utero-placental blood flow and is therefore a sign of a healthy pregnancy outcome (315).

Another explanation for this discrepancy could be a reduced maternal zinc status because iron and zinc competes in the body with one another for the same binding sites. In other words, the higher the body iron, the lower the body zinc and vice versa. As maternal zinc deficiency is already common, iron supplements can reduce it even further leading to even more prominent zinc deficiency and problems associated with it (115, 312). Whatever the case, it is important to remember that no nutrient works in the body in isolation, they always work as a team. Therefore, it is best not to take high doses of one dietary supplements alone, at least on long term, as it is bound to lead to deficiencies of the others. The most sensible idea is to get in touch with a qualified nutrition consultant or a doctor who is expert in nutritional medicine.

Manganese:
Maternal manganese deficiency in animal studies is linked with a

variety of skeletal malformations including enlarged hock joints, crooked and shortened legs and defective cartilage formations (316). In humans, maternal manganese deficiency has been associated with spina bifida, anencephaly, hydrocephalus and malformed limbs (317).

Toxic excesses:
Not only nutritional deficiencies but also toxic excesses can harm the unborn child in a variety of ways. Let's look first at alcohol.

Alcohol:
Though a moderate alcohol consumption makes us merry and is generally good for our health, anyone planning to get pregnant should drink no alcohol at all because it has both mutagenic (damages the gentic code) and teratogenic (damages the unborn foetus) properties. As such, it is able to damage the growing foetus in varying degrees throughout the whole pregnancy which can occur at the very earliest, as well as at the very lowest level of intake. In fact, alcohol-induced foetal damage has been linked with every form of drinking pattern, from heavy drinking to intermittent social drinking i.e. by consuming not more than one or two drinks in most days during pregnancy. So-called 'binge drinking' prior to pregnancy recognition is particularly dangerous because the most rapid period of the foetal organ formation occurs at the very earliest weeks after gestation. Considering that alcohol is a powerful teratogen, it has an ability to damage the growing foetus irreversibly leading to all types of mental and physical malformations (17).

However, alcohol-induced foetal damage tends to be devided in two distinct categories. At one end of the spectrum are children born to mothers who have been drinking heavily during pregnancy. These children are diagnosed as suffering from Foetal Alcohol Syndrome (FAS) which is recognised by strange flattened facial features. Also, the majority of children with FAS are born with a variety of heart, musculoskeletal and nervous system abnormalities. Many may also suffer from varying degrees of mental deficiency. In fact, it has been estimated that maternal alcoholism is responsible for at least 10% of all infant malformations ranging from serious heart and musculoskeletal defects to mental handicap (17).

At the other end of the spectrum are the children who lack these facial characteristics associated with FAS but who nevertheless suffer from subtle mental deficiencies due to the fact that even a low-level maternal alcohol intake can have the most insidious effect on the foetal brain growth and development. Infants born to mothers who have been drinking socially during pregnancy are not only born with a relatively small brain but the teratogenic effect of alcohol reduces the number of brain neurons and alters their distribution (17).

This affliction is known as Foetal Alcohol Effects (FAE). Ever increasing research evidence has shown that children with FAE suffer far more frequently from mental health problems than those born to mothers who did not drink whilst pregnant. These are known to include: poor co-ordination and organisations skills, impulsiveness, distractibility, learning disabilities, lowered IQ scores and childhood hyperactivity. Also, the majority of infants born to mothers who have been drinking socially during pregnancy are lighter at birth than children born to non-drinkers (17).

Alcohol consumption also leads to nutritional deficiencies of which alcohol-induced zinc and folic acid depletion are particularly well documented (17). Considering the dangers associated with low maternal folic acid and zinc status, all the more of a reason why the wuman should not drink alcohol whilst pregant. In males, zinc deficiency is known to lead to a reduced sperm count, slow sperm motility and a malformed sperm (115). Also, because alcohol has mutagenic properties, the male should avoid alcohol for about four months before planned conception whilst his sperm is still maturing. To make sure that the infant has the best start in life, Foresight recommends that both future parents should avoid alcohol for about four months before conception and the future mother should not drink any alcohol at all whist she is expecting (308, 309)

Cigarettes:
Cigarettes are not only associated with the development of cancer but like alcohol, they have both mutagenic and teratogenic properties. The reason why maternal cigarette smoking is dangerous for the unborn is because it does not only depress and disorganise the early foetal cell replication process but also hinders protein synthesis. It is therefore not suprising that ever increasing research evidence is linking maternal cigatte smoking with all kinds of birth malformations (18). For example, a study conducted among 10,523 health professionals found that infant malformations increased by 29% among those who were smoking cigarettes whilst pregnant compared to non-smokers. These included harelip, cleft palate and a wide variety of heart, digestive and central nervous system abnormalities (318). Others have found that children born to mothers have been smoking cigarettes whilst pregnant, suffer far more frequently from skin diseases, respiratory disorders and allergies compared to children born to mothers who did not smoke whilst expecting (18).

Furthermore, ever increasing number of research studies have reported that children born to mothers who were smoking cigarettes whilst pregnant, are far more likely to suffer from increased intellectual impairment and/or behavioural abnormalities compared to those born to non-smokers. These are known to include: short attention span, childhood hyperactivity, learning disabilities and malfunctions in both mental and intellectual development (18). Others have found that children born to mothers who have been smoking whilst expecting are far more likely to become juvenile delinquents compared to those born to mothers who did not smoke whilst pregnant (319).

As far as males are concerned, smoking is associated with a low sperm count, slow sperm motility and a malformed sperm (18). The latter was also proven using animal experiments. When male mice were exposed to nicotine and then coupled with perfectly healthy female dams, the pups were born with severe limb and other congenital malformations (320). If nothing else, at least this study highlights the fact that regardless of whether the female is gleaming with health, a malformed sperm produces malformed offspring. Not only that but some findings indicate that paternal cigarette smoking, by damaging the sperm, may be resposible for a child developing cancer in later life (321).

After years of assuming that the mother-to-be is only one responsible for the health of the unborn, a campaign similar to Foresight's, entitled 'Men Have Babies Too', has been established in America (322). It points out that smoking, drinking and environmental factors which, in the past, only pregnant women have been told to be aware of, can have a potentially harmful effect on the male sperm and hence on the unborn child. Besides reducing the changes of conception, a damaged sperm is a frequent cause for both miscarriages and foetal malformations. This being the case, guidelines are being drawn in the United States to encourage prospective fathers to go through a detoxification program before starting a family. First of all, men are advised to give up alcohol and cigarettes for at least four months before planned conception. Furthermore that this cleansing process should be accompanied by a diet rich in fresh fruit and vegetables including vitamin and mineral supplements. In special cases, the potential father may even be advised to give up his job for a period of time if it involves working in toxic atmosphere such as a paint shop or other high-risk occupations including some new-tech industries such as computing where special fluids are used for servicing and repairs. Dr Devra Lee Davis, a toxicologist, who is at the centre of the campaign, said: "For too long we've focused solely on mothers and what they should do to steer clear of toxic chemicals that cause birth defects. The importance of the father in making healthy babies has been under-appreciated. People only seem to start thinking about their unborn baby's health when they find out there is a child on the way. It should be a much longer process of planning and it should involve both partners, not just mother. We are not trying to scare men into believing that if they have drunk and smoked all their lives, or taken noxious substances, or worked in the chemical factory, they will father deformed children. It does not work like that. New sperm is produced all the time. But, in my view, men thinking about starting a family should begin preparations at least four months before they hope to start trying for a baby. They should give up all the obvious things, like cigarettes and drink, and they should take medical advice on healthy diet with good vitamin balance" (322). This is precisely what Foresight has been advocating for over twenty years (308, 309).

Synthetic food additives:

At least in animal studies, some synthetic food additives have been found to have either carcinogenic (cancer producing) mutagenic (damaging the gentic code) and/or teratogenic (damaging the unborn foetus) properties (126,211). For example, when a food additive amaranth (E123) was fed to rats, it led to cancer, stillbirths, sterility and early foetal deaths. Also ponceau (E124), red 2G (128), caramels (E150), brown FK (154) and sulphites (E220-227) were found to act as a mutagen and erythrosine (E127), nitrates (E249-E252), butylated hydroxyanisole (E320) and butylated hydroxytoluene (E321) were associated with both mutagenic and carcinogenic properties. Furthermore, artificial sweeteners such as saccharin and aspartame have been linked with both cancer and foetal malformations (126, 211). Therefore, just to be on the safe side, Foresight recommends that both prospective parents ought to avoid eating foods that contain synthetic food additives about four months before conception takes place and the future mother whilst she is expecting (308, 309).

Pesticide residues:

The London Food Commission lists 35 pesticides that have been linked in animal studies with adverse reproductive effects. These are known to include aldrin, benomyl, captan, carbaryl, dieldrin, dinoseb, ioxynil, maneb and paraquat (211). I have already mentioned that the mutagenic effect of pesticides became particularly noticeable when American servicemen who were exposed during the Vietnam war to a defoliant called Agent Orange, fathered children with an unusually high number of birth defects. Also that their female partners suffered from high rates of miscarriage and stillbirths (206). Yet again, to be on the safe side, Foresight recommends that it is best for both future parents to eat organically grown produce. Not only because they are free from pesticide residues but also because they have a far higher mineral content compared to the commercially grown variety (308, 309).

Genito-urinary infections:
Whilst the classical veneral diseases such as syphilis and gonorrhea have declined due to early detection and treatment, their place has been taken by other sexually transmitted infections of which the most widely spread is chlamydia trachomatis. The trouble with clamydia is that it carries hardly any symptoms, so that the infection can go undetected for a long time, only becoming noticeable when it has reached the Fallopian tubes where it manifests itself as pelvic inflammatory disease (PID) which is one of the main causes of female infertility (323). It is estimated that chlamydia affects one in five sexually active women in Britain. Furthermore, that it may be responsible for up to one third of all female infertility cases. If indentified at an early stage, the infection can be easily cured with antibiotic medication. For example in Europe, where chlamydial screening is commonplace, it has led to a marked fall in the number of women suffering from infertility problems (324).

Yet another trouble with chlamydial infection is that babies delivered through a chlamydia-infected birth canal may develop 'chlamydial infection' during the delivery which can be responsible for the following complications: inflammation of the eye (inclusion conjunctivitis) and ear (otitis media), lung infection (pneumonitis), gastroenteritis and an 'unspecified viral disease' (323). Considering the dangers associated with chlamydial and other genitourinary infections, Foresight recommends that both future parents have a check-up at a Genitourinary Medicine Clinic (308, 309).

Heavy metal contamination:
When Dr Neil Ward and his team studied 37 placental element levels of 100 obstetrically normal births, they found that the higher the mother's placental cadmium and/or lead level, the smaller the baby's head circumference and the lighter the infant was at birth. As both lead

and cadmium have the ability to chelate zinc from the body chemistry, the results showed that the mothers with the smallest babies had the lowest zinc status (325). Besides lead and cadmium, also other heavy metals such as aluminium, mercury and an excess of copper can harm the unborn child in a variety of ways. For this reason Foresight always recommends that both prospective parents should have their hair analysed before starting a family (308, 309).

Hair-mineral analysis:
Until recently, the recognition and consequent treatment of heavy metal contamination, as well as trace- and macromineral deficieny, has been hindered by a lack of reliable diagnostic techniques. Although blood, sweat and urine have been used these have been found to be ineffective in detecting a long- term exposure because the body fluids are in a constant state of flux, thereby reflecting only a very recent exposure of some hours or days (326-328).

However, since the development of modern laboratory techniques such as atomic absorption spectometry and neutron activation analysis, mineral concentrations can now be measured from the smallest of samples with the greatest of accuracy (328-332). Particularly since the introduction of the inductively coupled plasma mass spectometry (ICP-MS) system which has multi-detection capacity, hair tissue analysis has become the diagnostic tool of choice. Not only does it have the ability to measure toxic metals but at the same time it is able to give a clear indication of whole body's mineral status (329-331).

The advantages of hair tissue analysis over other diagnostic samples are as follows; First, the sample collection is non- invasive. Second, analytical methods are relatively easy as minerals in the hair are higher compared to other tissue measurements. Third, mineral concentrations in the hair are not subject to rapid fluctuations due to diet and other variables, therefore reflecting a long-term nutritional status (329, 332).

Hair mineral analysis has had in the past a rather doubtful reputation because different laboratories tended to use different sample preparations which obviously affected the outcome. However, since most reputable laboratories are currently using similar preparation and digestion processes, the results are becoming more identical. Neverthless, it is unlikely that the results between laboratories will ever be excactly alike because each machine tends to have its own unique level of sensitivity. Therefore, in order to avoid fluctuations in comparing results, it is always best to use the same laboratory instrument (329).

In cases where the hair-test analysis shows that toxic metals are above the recommended threshold, Foresight advises an individually tailored cleansing programme which may include, besides essential minerals, also vitamin C and/or garlic which have the ability to cleanse toxic metals from the body chemistry. If the results show that essential minerals are low, Foresight recommends appropriate supplements. This programme is given for a stated period when the hair will be re-tested. In cases where the results have not yet reached the levels required for a healthy foetal development, supplements are either repeated, or adjusted, until hair-tissue analysis is compatible with the optimum health of the future infant (308, 309).

These are just a few examples on which Foresight bases its preconception care work. It covers the most vulnerable time of the future baby's life when harmful influences can inflict permanent damage on the newborn. In other words, their work bridges the most vital period between existing Family Planning and Ante-natal Services - a gap left currently wide open within the National Health Service.

By using this simple nutritional approach, Foresight has helped literally thousands of couples to achieve a healthy pregnancy. Their success has been quite staggering. For example, one of their research experiments conducted by Dr Neil Ward at the Surrey University Chemistry Department, involving 367 couples with a previous history of reproductive failures, shows that Foresight's preconception care programme is not only effective but also scientifically sound. Of the 367 couples taking part, 136 suffered from infertility problems, 139 had had from one to five previous miscarriages and 45 had babies born with a low birth weight. In addition, 11 couples had given birth to a stillborn child and a further 7 had a child born malformed. Since the enrolment and within the timescale of the study, 327 women gave birth. In contrast to the couples' previous experiences, there were no miscarriages and every baby was born perfectly healthy and with a normal birth weight (333).

Low birth weight babies:
Mortality of very low birth weight babies has declined due to modern paediatric care. Though this is good news, ever increasing research evidence has found that the smaller the baby at birth the more likely he will suffer from different handicaps if he survives (334). These are known to include cerebral palsy (335, 336), impaired lung function (337), blindness, deafness, autism and epilepsy (338). Also, even slightly underweight babies at birth are more likely to suffer from learning disabilities, co-ordination problems, hyperactivity and other behavioural disorders compared to children born with a normal weight (339-345).

Also retrospective studies have found that low-birth weight infants, when they mature, are far more prone to health complications compared to those born with a normal weight. Evidence to that effect was carefully gathered together by Professor Barker and his colleagues from old medical records of 16,000 people born in Hertfordshire between 1911 and 1930. The results show that a low birth weight is associated in later life with the development of heart disease (346-349), increased cholesterol levels (350), high blood pressure (351, 352) and mature onset diabetes (353, 354). As references indicate, also other researches have come independently to the same conclusions.

According to the press, Britain shares with Albania one of the worst records in Europe for producing seriously underweight babies. In fact, seven per cent of infants born in England and Wales are classified as 'low birth weight'. Also, 50,000 babies are born each year which can only survive with the help of intensive care, sometimes lasting for months and costing £900 a day. If these poor creatures manage to live, this puts them at a high risk of mental handicap, deafness, cerebral palsy, epilepsy and autism (355).

Not that long ago the Earl Baldwin of Bewdley delivered a speech in the House of Lords of which I only cite a few extracts: "In the realm of reproductive health Professor Barker in Southampton has been showing that malnutrition in the womb can affect health in later life. But few people know of the pioneering work of a small organisation called Foresight, which for years has been targeting the health of couples before conception. In this country one quarter of all pregnancies ends in miscarriage, one baby in 11 is born prematurely, one in 17 is malformed, to say nothing of those many couples who are unable to conceive at all. Foresight's doctors attend to the parents' diets, especially their micronutrient levels, to the possibility of toxic overload with lead or other substances, and to symptom-less genito- urinary infections. In a recent uncontrolled trial involving 367 couples, 89 per cent of the women became pregnant soon after, and every one of the 327 children was born healthy and without problems, including to a high proportion to parents who had previously suffered from infertility or other difficulties. When you consider all that is involved in vitro fertilisation you would think that some encouragement might be given to a low-cost alternative, instead of the demand that Foresight should fund and conduct a double-blind trial which by nature of the treatment is an impossibility" (356).

Considering that one in six British couples has difficulty in conceiving, one baby in four is miscarried, one in 73 is stillborn or suffers from neonatal death, one in 17 has a malformation, many requiring surgery, and one in 11 are born so early that only intensive care might be able to save their lives, it is not only grazy but also highly unethical even to suggest that Foresight ought to conduct double-blind experiments to prove that this misery can be prevented by doing nothing else but eating wholesome foods and, if appropriate, taking harmless nutritional supplements. Particularly because by using this simple nutritional approach, which incidently covers the most vulnerable time of the baby's life when harmful influences can inflict permanent damage on the unborn – a cap left currently wide open within the National Health Service, Foresight has already helped literally thousands of couples to achieve a healthy pregnancy outcome. One wonders how much longer we have to wait until Foresight's pre-conception work gets the recognition it truly deserves?

The most distressing aspect of this whole situation is that we don't even seem to be satisfied with destroying our own health, sanity and reproductive capacity with the non-nutritious foods we eat, we want the whole world to suffer from the same faith. In fact, even increasing evidence has already established a dramatic trend of globalisation in countries which have adopted a Western-style diet and a paralell globalisation of associated diseases. Countries which have adopted Western foods, cancer deaths are already soaring which hardly knew the disease a few years ago. Similarly heart disease, also linked to inadequate diet, is increasing rapidly in developing countries because their population has adopted our unhealthy eating habits. The same with obesity and diabetes (357). Have we no shame?

I would like to finish this chapter citing a few verses from a brilliant poem by Joseph Malines entitled "The Ambulance down in the Valley" which describes to perfection the futility associated with our modern 'health-care' system.

> Twas a dangerous cliff, as they freely confessed
> though to walk near its crest was pleasant.
> But over its edge there slipped a duke and many a peasant.
> So the people said something would have to be done,
> but their project did not tally;
> Some said, 'Put a fence round the edge of the cliff'
> Some 'An ambulance down in the valley'.
> Then an old man remarked, 'It is marvel to me,
> that people give far more attention,
> to repairing results than stopping the cause,
> when they much better aim at prevention.
> Let us stop its source all this mischief' cried he,
> Come neighbours and friends, let us rally.
> If the cliff we will fence, we might almost dispense
> with the ambulance down in the valley'.

To build that fence and almost dispense with that ambulance down in the valley is the easiest thing in the world. All we have to do is eat a balanced diet prepared from organic produce. Drink moderately and enjoy ourselves. Kippis!

CHAPTER 10
THE NEW MILLENNIUM

A recent United Nations's survey 'Global Environmental Outlook 2000' points out that our planet is facing at the moment a string of full-scale catastrophies which are threatening our world and survival. The survey, which was compiled by 200 eminent scientists from 50 countries, found the following: Nearly 80% of the world's rainforests, the planet's 'green lungs' and vital habitats for wild-life, have been destroyed for timber and agriculture. Also other forests are dying at an alarming rate due to traffic and industrial pollution. Directly due to man-made pollution, already a quarter of world's mammals and 11% of bird species are at serious risk of extinction. The same with marine life which is rapidly being poisoned by agricultural and industrial effluent.

The survey also estimated that by 2025 there will be up to a billion cars on the roads resulting in traffic pollution which, besides doing a great deal of harm to our ecosystem, will be responsible for several million human deaths each year. The same with ever increasing pesticide pollution. Furthermore, that waste levels in industrial countries are increasing approximately by 30% every ten years, most ending up in rubbish tips (358).

Not only are we poisoning our planet and ourselves with industrial, traffic and agricultural effluent but at the same time, largely by burning fossil fuels, we are responsible for global warming which has already led to extreme weather conditions such as severe droughts in some parts of the world and excessive flooding in others. In fact, it is estimated that if we allow the atmospheric warming to continue at its present rate, the speed in which ice glaciers are melting, most low-lying coastal areas and land masses will be disappearing under the sea within the next hundred years.

But nature is no fool, it hits back. It is highly arrogant even to imagine that we can dominate our planet to suit our greed. The wide use of agrochemicals has already resulted in thousands of weeds and pests developing resistance. The same with excessive use of antibiotics which has led to the development of antibiotic-resistant bacteria against which no known antibiotics can prevail. Now we are tinkering with genetically modified crops. Though this is yet at its early stage, it is becoming already apparent that this man-made technology will end up as another ecological disaster. Also falling sperm counts, including infertility, perhaps the most sensitive barometer of animal and human destruction, can be laid at the door of modern chemical industries.

It is even more absurd to imagine that the world is a cycle in which riches circulate forever. Because of our greed, we are not only in process of destroying the soil, forests, waterways and the air on which all our living systems depend but also squandering our unrenewable energy resources such as coal, oil and natural gas on which our modern industries rely. Only waste and rubbish are thriving.

As modern chemical industries are inevitably responsible for most of our global destruction, it is obvious that the only way to save our planet and consequently the human race is to create an economy which is less dependent on these highly destructive practices. According to Edward Goldsmith, the editor of The Ecologist (359): "The environmental problems we face today, such as destruction of the world's forests, the drainage of its wetlands, the pollution of its groundwaters, rivers, estuaries, seas; the erosion, campaction and desertification of its agricultural lands, the chemicalisation of just about everything, and of course global climate change, are not unrelated. They form a veritable syndrome, and they are the inevitable consequences of the policies we apply, all of which are designed to contribute to the overriding policy of promoting the massive, uncontrolled, economic development that we identify with progress. Unfortunately we believe quasi-religiously in economic development.

Underlying the world-view of this secular religion is the fundamental assumption that the world is badly designed. God did a bad job, and it is incumbent on man, armed as he is with all his science, technology, industry and free trade, to transform it in accordance with his vastly superior design. To a truly religious person this dogma must be the ultimate blasphemy; yet few people see it that way. Nearly everyone today seems to accept the preposterous view that modern man is actually 'improving' the world - making a better place to live in – against, I might add, all evidence to the contrary that is accumulating by the minute...

It is quite clear that today there are no cosmetic solutions to our problems. Of all today's social and ecological trends lead to catastrophe, quite obviously the only responsible course of action is to reverse these trends and reverse them very quickly indeed. If today's policy is to create a global economy totally controlled by vast, uncontrollable and irresponsible transnational corporations catering for the world market, we must instead create a network of loosely connected local ecologies, largely in the hands of small and medium companies that are integral parts of local communities and societies, and for whom they feel deeply responsible. It is only in this way that we can reduce the impact of our economic activities on an environment that cannot sustain the present impact – an impact that we are still busily trying to increase by globalising the economy and making it ever more dependent on the use of highly destructive new technologies such as genetic engineering.

It is only this way that we can conceivably provide people with jobs or other means of assuring their livelihood, for it is the small and medium companies that provide the bulk of available jobs – the transnationals, in spite of all their hype, providing but an insignificant proportion of those that are today available. What is more, it is only in this way that we can create the economic infrastructure for renewed family and community life..." (359).

The irreparable impact of modern technologies have affected most sections of our life. In medicine it has led to an epidemic of iatrogenic (treatment induced) diseases as an ever-increasing number of individuals are incapacitated or die from the effects of prescribed medication.

The reason why modern medicines are so dangerous for our health is because their initial testing for toxicity has been performed by using animal experiments. Not only that these 'tests' are highly misleading and unscientific, they also inflict an enormous cruelty and suffering to animals.

If for no other reason except to save our own health and sanity, we have got to demand that animal experiments are made illegal by law. Mark my words, it will not take long before the world's medical profession will agree that vivisection has been the biggest folly in medical history!

I should like to end my writing with words inspired by Chief Seattle, to whom I dedicated this book: "We know that the white man does not understand our ways. One portion of land is the same to him as the next, for he is a stranger who comes in the night and takes from the land whatever he needs. The earth is not his brother, but his enemy, and when he has conquered it, he moves on. He leaves his fathers' grave behind and kidnaps the earth from his children. His appetite will devour the earth and leave only a desert. When all the beasts are slaughtered, the wild horses tamed, the secret corners of the forests heavy with the scent of many men and the view of the ripe hills blotted by talking wires, where is the thicket? Gone. Where is the eagle? Gone. And what it is to say goodbye to the swift and the hunt, the end of living and the beginning of survival? We might understand if we knew what the white man dreams, what hopes he describes to his children in long winter nights, what vision he burns onto their eyes so that they will wish for tomorrow. I pray they are told that man did not weave the web of life; he is merely a strand in it. Whatever befalls the earth, befalls the children of earth. Whatever he does to the web, he does it to himself" (360). Amen.

REFERENCES

1. Gregory JR, et al: National Diet and Nutrition Survey: Children aged 1 ¹/₂-4 ¹/₂ years. Volume 1: Report of the Diet and Nutrition Survey, 1995. HMSO Publications, PO Box 276, London SW8 5DT

2. Doyle W, et al: Nutritional status of schoolchildren in inner city area. Arch Dis Child, 70: 376-381, 1994

3. Wenlock RW, et al: The Diets of British Schoolchildren: A preliminary report of nutritional analysis of a nationwide survey of British schoolchildren, April, 1986 HMSO Publications,

4. Teenage Eating Habits: A summary of a survey carried out by the National Dairy Council in conjunction with Youth Express Newspaper, NDC, 5-7 John Princes Street, London W1M 0AP, UK. 1995.

5. Bull NC: Dietary habits of 15 to 25 year-olds. Applied Nutrition 39A, suppl.1: 1-68,1985.

6. Ewes A, et al: Changes in the diets of university students over a six-year period (1986-1991). J Human Nutr and Diet, 7:363-376, 1994

7. Gregory, J, et al: The Dietary and Nutritional Survey of British Adults, HMSO Publications, 1990

8. Ministry of Agriculture, Fisheries and Food Household Food Consumption and Expenditure Survey, 1991 HMSO Publications, 1992

9. MAFF (1993) National Food Survey, HMSO Publications, 1994

10. MAFF (1996) National Food Survey, HMSO Publications, 1997

11. Breeze E, et al: Health Survey for England 1992. HMSO Publications, 1994

12. RCGP, OPCS 'Morbidity Statistics from General Practice: Fourth national study 1992-93', HMSO Publications, 1995

13. Muldoon MF, Manuck SB, Matthews KA: Lowering cholesterol concentration and mortality: A quantitive review of primary prevention trials. Br Med J, 301:309-314, 1990

14. Engelberg H: Low serum cholesterol and suicide. Lancet, 339: 727-729,1992

15. Ravnskov U: Cholesterol lowering trials in coronary heart disease: frequency in citation and outcome. Lancet, 305: 15-19, 1992

16. Laurance J: Scientists say that bottle of wine a day is the key to longer life. The Times, 5th May, 1995

17. Tuormaa TE: The adverse effects of alcohol on reproduction. J Nutr & Environ Med, 6 (4): 379-391,1996

18. Tuormaa TE: The adverse effects of tobacco smoking on reproduction and health: A review from the literature. Nutrition and Health, 10: 105-120, 1995

19. Greden JF: Anxiety and caffeinism: a diagnostic dilemma. Am J Psychiatry, 131: 1089-1092, 1974

20. Horrobin DF: Essential fatty acids: A review. In: Clinical Uses of Essential Fatty Asids. Ed: D.F. Horrobin, Eden Press Inc, 1982

21. Effective Nutritional Medicine: The Application of Nutrition to Major Health Problems. Published by The British Society of Allergy and Environmental Medicine with the British Society for Nutritional Medicine, PO Box 7, Knighton LD7 1WT, UK. 1995

22. Sanders TAB, et al: The comparison of the influence on plasma lipids and platelet function of supplements of w3 and w6 polyunsaturated fatty acids. Br J Nutr, 50: 521-530, 1983

23. Singer P, et al: Influence on serum lipids, lipoproteins and blood pressure of mackarel and herring diet in patients with type of IV and V hyperlipoproteinemia. Artherosclerosis, 56 (1): 111-118, 1985

24. Simons LA, et al: On the effects of dietary n-3 fatty acids (MaxEPA) on plasma lipids and lipoproteins in patients with hyperlipidemia. Atherosclerosis, 54: 75-88, 1985

25. Macdonald MC, et al: Dietary linoleic acid and salt-induced hypertension. Canad J Physiol, 59: 872-875, 1981

26. Jacono JM, et al: The role of dietary essential fatty acids and prostaglandins in reducing blood pressure. Progr Lipid Res, 20: 571-574, 1982

27. Woodcock BE, et al: Beneficial effects of fish oil on blood viscosity in peripheral vascular disease. Br Med J, 288: 592-594, 1984

28. Kemoff PBA, et al: Antithrombotic potential of dihomo-gamma linolenic acid in man. Br Med J, 2: 1441, 1977

29. Darcet P, et al: Effects of a diet enriched with gamma linoleic acid on PUFA metabolism and platelet aggregation in elderly men. Ann Nutr Aliment, 34: 277-290, 1980

30. Fisher JM, et al: Effects of prostaglandins and their precursors in some tests of hemostatic function. Progr Lipid Res, 20: 799-806, 1982

31. Christie SBM, et al: Observations on the performance of a standard excercise test by claudicans taking gamma-linolenic acid. J Artheroscler Res, 8: 83-90, 1978

32. Saynor R, et al: The long-term effect of dietary supplementation with fish lipid concentrate on serum lipids, bleeding time, platelets and angina. Atherosclerosis 50: 3-10, 1984

33. Zurier RB, et al: Effects of prostaglandin E1 on adjuvant arthritis. Nature, 234: 304-305, 1971

34. Horrobin DF, et al: The nutritional regulation of T-lymphocyte function. Medical Hypotheses, 5: 969-985, 1979

35. Horrobin DF: Regulation of prostaglandin biosynthesis: negative feedback mechanisms and the selective control of formation of 1 and 2 series prostaglandins: relevance to inflammation and immunity. Medical Hypotheses, 6: 687-709, 1980

36. Brush MG: Evening primrose oil (Efamol) in the treatment of the premenstrual syndrome. International Efamol Conference, London, November, 1981

37. Lovell CR, et al: Treatment of atopic eczema with evening primrose oil. Lancet, i: 278,1981

38. Dworkin RH: Linoleic acid and multiple sclerosis. Lancet, i: 1153-1154, 1981

39. Horrobin DF and Manku MS: Possible role of prostaglandins E1 in the affective disorders and alcoholism. Br Med J, 1: 1363-1366, 1980

40. Horrobin DF: A biochemical basis for alcoholism and for alcohol-induced damage including fetal alcohol syndrome and cirrhosis: interference with essential fatty acid and prostaglandin metabolism. Med Hypoteses, 6: 929-942, 1980

41. Horrobin DF: Prostaglandins and schizophrenia: further discussion and evidence. Psychol Med, 8: 43-48, 1978

42. Horrobin DF: Schizophrenia: reconciliation of the dopamine, prostaglandin and opioid concepts and the role of the pineal. Lancet, i: 529-531, 1979

43. Horrobin DF, Glen AIM, Vaddadi K: The membrane hypothesis in schizophrenia. Schizophrenia Research,13: 195-207, 1994

44. Colquhoun V and Bunday S: A Lack of essential fatty acids as a possible cause of hyperactivity in children Med Hypotheses, 7: 681-686, 1981

45. Stevens LJ, et al: Essential fatty acid metabolism in boys with attention-deficit hyperactivity disorder. Am J Clin Nutr, 62: 761-768, 1995

46. Hawkes N: Margarine linked to breast cancer. The Times, 5th September, 1997

47. Willett WC, et al: Intake of trans fatty acids and risk of coronary heart disase among women. Lancet, 341: 581-585, 1993

48. Finn R: Letters to the Editor The Times, 24th May, 1994

49. Yudkin J: Pure, White and Deadly. Viking, 1986

50. Larsen H: Heart Disease: A Review. Int J Alt Compl Med, 14 (5): 9-10, 1996 Prevention: the golden rules. Int J Alt Compl Med, 14 (6): 9-10, 1996. Heart disease: conventional treatments. Int J Alt Compl Med, 14 (7): 9-10, 1996. Heart of the matter. Int J Alt Compl Med, 14 (8): 14-15, 1996

51. Duffy, SJ. et al: Treatment of hypertension with ascorbic acid. Lancet, 354:2048-2049. 1999

52. Rath M and Pauling L: Solution to the puzzle of human cardiovascular disease: its primary cause is ascorbate deficiency leading to the deposition of lipoprotein (a) and fibrinogen/fibrin in the vascular wall. J Orthomolecular Med, 6: 125-134, 1991

53. Stampfer MJ and Rimm EB: Epidemiologic evidence of vitamin E in prevention of cardiovascular disease. Am J Clin Nutr, Vol (suppl) 62: 1365S-1369S, 1995

54. Boushey CJ, et al: A quantitative assessment of plasma homocysteine as a risk factor for cardiovascular disease. JAMA, 274 (13): 1049-1057, 1995

55. Reusser ME and McCarron DA: Micronutrient effects on blood pressure regulation. Nutrition Reviews, 52 (11): 367-375,1994

56. Appel LJ, et al: Does supplementation of diet with 'fish oil' reduce blood pressure? Arch Int Med, 153: 1429-1438, 1993

57. Kendler BS: Garlic (Allium sativum) and onion (Allium cepa): a review of their relationship to cardiovascular disease. Preventive Med, 16: 670-685, 1987

58. Strong JP and McGill HR Jr: The natural history of coronary atherosclerosis. Am J Pathol, 40: 37-49, 1962

59. McNamara JJ, et al: Coronary artery heart disease in combat casualties in Vietnam. JAMA, 216: 1185-1187, 1971

60. Laurance J: Rapid rise in the number of cancer sufferes. The Times, 20th October, 1996

61. Higginson J: Environmental carcinogens. Cancer Supplement, 72: 971-977, 1993

62. Doll R: An overview of the epidemiological evidence linking diet and cancer. Proceedings of the Nutrition Society, 49: 119-131, 1990

63. Seely S and Horrobin DF: Diet and breast cancer: The possible connection with sugar consumption. Med Hypotheses, 11 (3): 319-327, 1983

64. Sanchez A, et al: The role of sugars in human neutrophilic phagocytosis. Am J Clin Nutr, 26: 180-184, 1973

65. Block G: Fruits, vegetables and cancer prevention: a review from the epidemio logical evidence. Nutrition and Cancer, 18: 1-29, 1992

66. Thurnham DI: Chemical aspects and biological mechanism of anticancer nutrients in plant foods. In: Waldron KV, et al (eds) Food and Cancer Prevention: Chemical and Biological Aspects, pp 109-118 Cambridge, Royal Society of Chemistry, 1993

67. Neil K: Living food revolution. J Optimum Nutr, 8 (2): 28-35, 1995

68. Goodman S: Nutrition and Cancer – State of the Art. Green Library Publications, 1995

69. Murray I: Cancer threat is on the increase. The Times, 25th June, 1997

70. Hoffer A: A Guide to Eating Well for Pure Health: Hoffer's Laws of Natural Nutrition. Quarry Press Inc, PO Box 1061, Kingston, Ontario K7L 4Y5, 1996

71. MIND Information: Mental Health Statistics, MIND Publications, UK, 1994

72. Laurance J: One adult in seven has mental disorder. The Times, 15th December, 1994

73. Kennedy D: Mental illness 'will strike 40% of children'. The Times, 2nd December, 1996

74. Neurotransmitters and CNS Disease: A Lancet Review: First published in consecutive issues, Oct. 23 to Dec.18, 1982

75. Harris S: Hyperinsulinism and dysinsulinism. J Am Med Assoc, 83:729-733, 1924

76. Thorn GW, et al: A comparison of the metabolic effects of isocaloric meals of varying composition with special reference to the prevention of post-prandial hypoglycaemic symptoms. Ann Int Med, 18 (6): 913-919, 1943

77. Lesser M: Nutrition & Vitamin Therapy: The Dietary Treatment of Mental and Emotional Ill-health. Thorsons, UK, 1980

78. Budd M: Low Blood Sugar (Hypoglycaemia) – The 20th Century Epidemic? Thorsons, UK, 1981

79. Airola P: Hypoglycaemia: A Better Approach. Health Plus Publishers, Phoenix, Arizona, US, 1977

80. Food Intolerance and Food Adversion – A Joint Report of the Royal College of Physicians and the British Nutritional Foundation. Royal College of Physicians, 18 (2), April, 1984

81. Virkkunen M and Huttunen MO: Evidence for abnormal glucose tolerance test among habitually violent offenders. Neurophysiology, 8: 30-34, 1982

82. Virkkunen M: Reactive hypoglycaemic tendency among habitually violent offenders: A further study by means of the glucose tolerance test. Neurophysiology, 8: 35-40, 1982

83. Virkkunen M: Insulin secretion during the glucose tolerance test in antisocial personality. Br J Psychiatry, 142: 598-604, 1983

84. Tuormaa TE: An Alternative to Psychiatry. The Book Guild Ltd, UK, 1991.

85. Schauss AG: Nutrition and behavior: Complex inter-disciplinary research. Nutrition and Health, 3: 9-37, 1984

86. Carney MWP: Neuropsychiatric disorders associated with nutritional deficiencies: Incidence and therapeutic implications. CNS Drugs: 3 (4): 279-290, 1995

87. Pfeiffer CC: Mental and Elemental Nutrients. Keats Publishing Inc, New Canaan, Connecticut, 1975

88. Davies S and Stewart A: Nutritional Medicine: The drug-free quide to better family health. Pan Books, 1987

89. Tolonen M: Vitamins and Minerals in Health and Nutrition. Ellis Horwood Series in Food Science and Technology, 1990

90. Word B, et al: A study of partial thiamine restriction in human volunteers. Am J Clin Nutr, 33: 848-861, 1980

91. Lonsdale D and Shamberger RD: Red cell transketolase as an indicator of nutritional deficiency. Am J Clin Nutr, 33: 205-211, 1980

92. Sterns RT and Price WR: Restricted riboflavin: within behavioral effects in humans. Am J Clin Nutr, 26 (2): 150-160, 1973

93. Carney MWP, et al: Thiamin, riboflavin and pyridoxine deficiency in psychiatric in-patients. Br J Psychiatry, 141: 271-272, 1982

94. Green RG: Subclinical pellagra. In: Orthomolecular Psychiatry, Eds: D Hawkins and L Pauling, W.H. Freeman and Co, San Fransisco, 1973

95. Nobbs BT: Pyridoxal phosphate in clinical depression. Lancet: i: 405-406, 1974

96. Stewart TW, et al: Low B6 levels in depressed out-patients. Biol Psychiatry, 19: 613-616, 1984

97. Carney MWP, et al: Thiamine and pyridoxine lack in newly admitted psychiatric patients. Br J Psychiatry, 135: 249-254, 1979

98. Carney MWP: Serum folate levels in 423 psychiatric patients. Br Med J, 4: 512-516, 1967

99. Reynolds EH, et al: Folate deficiency in depressive illness. Br J Psychiatry, 117: 287-292, 1970

100. Thornton WE: Folic acid, mental function and dietary habits. J Clin Psychiatry, 39: 315-322, 1978

101. Botez MI and Reynolds EH (Eds): Folic acid in Neurology, Psychiatry and Internal Medicine, Raven Press, 1979

102. Ghadirian AM, et al: Folic acid deficiency and depression. Psychosomatics, 21(11):926-929, 1980

103. Shorvon SD, et al: The neuropsychiatry of megaloplastic anaemia. Br Med J, 281:1036-1038, 1980

104. Gray GE and Leong GB: Serum folate levels in U.S. psychiatric in-patients. J Clin Psychiatry, 47: 98-99, 1986

105. Crellin R, et al: Folate and psychiatric disorder: clinical potential. Drugs, 45: 623-636, 1993

106. Sneath P, et al: Folate status in a geriatric population and its relation to dementia. Age Ageing, 2: 177-182,1973

107. Shaw DM, et al: Senile dementia and nutrition. Br Med J, 281: 792-793, 1984

108. Hunter R, et al: Serum B12 and folate concentrations in mental patients. Br J Psychiatry, 113: 1291-1295, 1967

109. Kallstrom B and Nylof R: Vitamin B12 and folic acid in psychiatric disorders. Acta Psychiatr Scand, 43: 137-152,1969

110. Hallstrom T: Serum B12 and folate concentrations in mental patients. Acta Psychiatr Scand, 45: 19-36, 1969

111. Shulman R: Survey of vitamin B12 deficiency and psychiatric illness in an elderly psychiatric patients. Br J Psychiatry, 113: 241-251,1967

112. Evans DI, et al: Organic psychosis without anaemia of spinal cord symptoms on patients with vitamin B12 deficiency. Am J Psychiatry, 140: 218-220, 1983

113. Kinsman RA and Hood J: Some behavioral effects of ascorbic acid deficiency. Am J Clin Nutr, 24: 455-467, 1971

114. Bryce-Smith D and Hodginson L: The Zinc Solution.Century Arrow, 1987

115. Tuormaa TE: Adverse effects of zinc deficiency. J of Orthomolecular Med, 10 (3&4): 149-164, 1995

116. Burnet FM: A possible role of zinc in pathology of dementia. Lancet, i:186-188, 1981

117. Webb TE and Oski FA: Behavioral status of young adolescents with iron deficiency anemia. J Special Education, 8 (2): 153-156, 1974

118. Pollitt R, et al: Behavioral effects of iron deficiency anemia in children. In: Iron Deficiency, Brain Chemistry and Behavior. Eds: R. Pollitt and L. Leibel, pp 195-204, Raven Press, New York,1982

119. Addy DP: Happiness is iron. Br Med J, 292: 1599, 1986

120. O'Leary J and Carter D: Heads accused of cover-up over classroom thugs. The Times, 2nd April, 1996

121. Bryce-Smith D: Environmental and chemical influences on behaviour and mentation. (The John Jeyes Lecture, Royal Society of Chemistry) Chem Soc Rev, 14: 93-123, 1986. Also a sligty expanded version; Int J Biosocial Res, 8 (2): 115-150, 1986

122. Bryce-Smith D: Behavioural effects of lead and other heavy metal pollutants. Chem Brit, 8 (6): 240-243, 1972

123. Bryce-Smith D: Crime and nourishment. Scientific and Medical Network Review, 59: 3-6, 1995

124. Tuormaa TE: The adverse effects of lead. J Nutr Med, 4 (4): 449-461,1994

125. Needleman HL, et al: Deficits on psycohologic and classroom performance of children with elevated dentine lead levels. New Engl J Med, 300: 689-695,1979

126. Tuormaa TE: Adverse effects of food additives on health: With a special emphasis on childhood hyperactivity. J Orthomol Med, 9 (4): 225-246,1994

127. Barnes B and Colquhoun I: Hyperactive Child, Attention Deficit Hyperactive Disorder: A practical self-help guide for parents. Thorsons, 1997

128. Egger J, et al: Controlled trial of oligoantigenic treatment in the hyperkinetic syndrome. Lancet, i: 540-545, 1985

129. Egger J, et al: Is migraine a food allergy? – A double-blind controlled trial of oligoantigenic diet treatment. Lancet, ii: 65-869, 1983

130. Feingold BF: Hyperkinesis and learning disabilities linked to artificial food flavors and colors. Am J Nutr, 75: 797-803, 1975

131. Feingold BF: Why Your Child is Hyperactive? Random House, New York,1975

132. Tuormaa TE: A brief review of the immune system and its function in relation to: post viral fatigue syndrome (M.E.), non-antibody mediated allergy, autoimmunity and immune deficiency. Nutrition and Health, 6 (1): 53-62,1988

133. Crook WG: Food additives and hyperactivity. Lancet, p 1128, 15 May, 1982

134. Crook WG: Can what a child eats make him dull, stupid or hyperactive? J Learn Disabil, 3: 13, 1980

135. Crook WG: Defined diets and hyperactivity. Presentation at N.I.H. Consensus Development Conference on Hyperactivity, Bethesda, Maryland, 14 January,1982

136. Randolp TG: Allergy as a causative factor of fatigue, irritability, and behavior problems in children. J Pediatr, 31: 560, 1947

137. Speer F: The allergic tension-fatigue syndrome. Pediatr Clin N Am, 1:1029, 1954

138. Rapp DJ: Does diet affect hyperactivity? J Learn Disabil, 11: 56-62,1978

139. Rapp DJ: Food additives and hyperactivity. Lancet, p1128, 15 May,1982

140. Rowe AH: Food Allergy. Springfield, Charles Thomas, 1972

141. Randolph TG: Human Ecology and Susceptibility to the Chemical Environment. Springfield, Charles Thomas, 1962

142. Speer F: Allergic-tension-fatigue in children. Ann Allergy, 12: 168 1954

143. Crook WG: Systemic manifestations due to allergy. Pediatrics, 27: 790, 1961

144. Swanson JM and Kinsbourne M: Food dyes impair performance of hyperactive children on a laboratory learning test. Science, 207: 1485-1487, 1980

145. Conners CK, et al: Food additives and hyperkinesis: a controlled double-blind laboratory experiment. Pediatrics, 58: 154-166,1976

146. Harley JP, et al: Hyperkinesis and food additives: Testing the Feingold hypothesis. Pediatrics, 61: 818-128, 1978

147. Rapp DJ: Allergies and the Hyperactive Child. Cornerstone Library, New York, 1980

148. O'Shea JA and Porter SF: Double-blind study of children with hyperkinetic syndrome treated with multi-allegen subclinically. J Learn Disabil, 14: 189-237, 1981

149. Bunday S and Colquhoun V: Why the lack of treatment for hyperactive children? J Nutr Med, 1: 361-363, 1990

150. Menzies IC: Disturbed children: The role of food and chemical sensitivities. Nutrition and Health, 3: 39-54, 1984

151. British National Formularly: A joint publication of the British Medical Association and the Royal Pharmaceutical Society, Number 30, September, 1995

152. Dobson R: More children given 'chemical cosh'. Independent on Sunday, 12th October, 1997

153. Breggin P: Robots on parade. What Doctors Don't Tell You, 10(5):12, 1999

154. Benton D and Roberts G: Effect of vitamin and mineral supplementation on intelligence of a sample of schoolchildren. Lancet, i: 140-143, 1988

155. Eysenck HJ: Raising I.Q. through vitamin and mineral supplementation: an introduction. In: Improvement of I.Q. and behaviour as a function of dietary supplementation; A symposium. Ed: HJ Eysenck and SBG Eysenck, Pergamon Press,1991

156. Steiner S: School rises up the table of the junk-food ban. The Times, 20th May,1999

157. Bluin AGA, et al: Teenage alcohol use among hyperactive children: A five year follow-up study. J Pediatric Psychology, 3 (4): 188-194, 1978

158. Wood D, et al: The prevalence of attention deficit disorder, residual type, or minimal brain dysfunction, in a population of male alcoholic patients. Am J Psychiatry, 140: 95-98, 1983

159. Weiss G, et al: Hyperactives as young adults: A controlled prospective ten-year follow up of 75 children. Arch Gen Psychiatry, 36: 675-681, 1979

160. Schoenthaler SJ: The effects of sugar on the treatment and control of antisocial behavior: A double-blind study of an incarcerated juvenile population. Int J Biosocial Res, 3 (1): 1-9, 1982

161. Schoenthaler SJ: Diet and crime; An empirical examination of the value of nutrition in the control and treatment of incarcerated juvenile offenders. Int J Biosocial Res, 4 (1): 25-39, 1983

162. Schoenthaler SJ: The Alabama diet-behavior program: An empirical evaluation at the Coosa Valley Regional Detention Centre. Int J Biosocial Res, 5 (2): 79-87,1983

163. Schoenthaler SJ: The Los Angeles Probation Department diet-behavior program: An empirical analysis of six institutional settings. Int J Biosocial Res, 5 (2): 88-98, 1983

164. Schoenthaler SJ: The Northern California diet-behavior program: An empirical examination of 3,000 incarcerated juveniles in Stanislaus County Juvenile Hall. Int J Biosocial Res, 5 (2): 99-106, 1983

165. Schauss AG: Diet, Crime and Delinquency. Parker House, Berkeley, California 94714, US, 1981

166. Schauss AG: Nutrition and behaviour. J Applied Nutr, 35 (1): 30-43, 1983

167. Reed B: Food, Teens and Behavior. Natural Press, PO Box 2107, Manitowoc, WI54220, 1983

168. Ford R: Vitamins may wean young offenders from diet of crime. The Times, 12th April, 1996

169. Ford R: Young are committing 13 crimes each minute. The Times, 26th July, 1997

170. Rippere V: The diet of psychiatric patients. Soc for Environ Therapy Newsletter, 2 (1) 4-7, 1992

171. Marks I and Lader M: Anxiety States (Anxiety Neurosis): A Review. J Nerv Ment Dis, 156 (1): 3-18,1973

172. Magarian GJ: Hyperventilation Syndromes: Infrequently recognized common expressions of anxiety and stress. Medicine, 61 (4): 219-236, 1982

173. Randolp TG and Moss RW: Allergies, your Hidden Enemy How the new field of Clinical Ecology can unravel the environmental causes of mental and physical illness. Thorsons, UK,1981

174. Mackarness R: Not All in the Mind, Pan Books, 1990

175. Howard LM and Wessley S: Psychiatry in the allergy clinic: the nature and management of patients with non-allergic symptoms. Clin Exp Allergy, 25: 503-514, 1995

176. Laurance J: Disease is in the mind for quarter of patients. The Times, 13th May,1995.

177. Neuroleptic Drugs, In: Rang HP and Dale MM: Pharmacology, Churchill Livingstone 499-512, 1987

178. Kanof PD and Greenland P: Brain histamine receptors as targets for anti depressants drugs. Nature, 272: 329-333, 1978

179. Mazurkiewicz-Kwilecki IM: Possible role of histamine in brain function: neurochemical, physiological, and pharmacological indications. Can J Physiol Pharmacol, 62: 709-714,1984

180. Mental Illness: Not All in the Mind; ION Mental Health Project publication, Ed: P Holford, ION, London SW15 2NU, UK, 1995

181. Rynaerson EH and Moersch FP: Neurological manifestations of hyper-insulinism and other hypoglycaemic states. J Am Med Assoc, 103 (16): 1196-1199, 1934

182. Wilder J: Psychological problems of hypoglycaemia. Am J Digest Dis, 10 (11): 428-435,1943

183. Landman HR and Sutherland RL: Incidence and significance of hypoglycaemia in unseleceted admissions to a psychosomatic service. Am J Digest Dis, pp 105-108, 1950

184. Salzer HM: Relative hypoglycaemia as a cause of neuro-psychiatric illness. J Nat Med Assoc, 58 (1): 12-17, 1966

185. Gorman JM, et al: Hypoglycaemia and panic attacks. Am J Psychiatry, 141 (1): 101-102, 1984

186. Grant ECG: Food allergies and migraine. Lancet, ii: 966-68, 1979

187. Monro J, Carini C, Brostoff J: Migraine is a food-allergic disease. Lancet, ii:719-21, 1984

188. Darlington LG, Ramsey NW, Mansfield JR: Placebo-controlled blind study of dietary manipulation in rheumatoid arthritis. Lancet, i: 236-238, 1986

189. Jones VA, et al: Food intolernace: a major factor in the pathogenesis of irritable bowel syndrome. Lancet, ii: 1115-17, 1982

190. Bentall R: The illness that defies diagnosis. The Times, 20th may, 1996

191. Osmond H and Hoffer A: Massive niacin treatment in schizophrenia. Lancet, pp316-320, 10 February,1962

192. Hoffer A and Walker M: Smart Nutrients: A Guide to Nutrients that can prevent and reverse Senility. Avery Publishing Group, Garden City, New York,1994

193. Peiffer CC: Mental Illness: The Nutrition Connection Holford P: Mental Health: The Nutrition Connection. ION Press, UK, 1996

194. Hall RCW, et al: Physical illness manifesting as psychiatric disease. Arch Gen Psychiatry, 37: 989-995, 1980

195. Birchall JD and Chappel JS: Aluminium, chemical physiolology and Alzheimer's disease. Lancet, ii: 1008-1010, 1988

196. Graves AB, et al: The association between aluminium-containing products and Alzheimer's disease. J Clin Epidemiol, 43 (1): 35-44, 1990

197. Wenk GI and Stemmer KL: Suboptimal dietary zinc increases aluminium accumulation in the rat brain. Brain Res, 288: 393-395, 1983

198. Bryce-Smith D: Aluminium and the blood-brain barrier. J Alt & Compl Med, June, 1989

199. Assault on the Mind. Published by Channel 4 Television, 124 Horseferry Road, London SW1P 2TX, 1998

200. Chaitow L: Amino Acids in Therapy: A Guide to the Therapeutic Application of Protein Constituents. Thorsons, 1985

201. Millard PH: Treatment for ageing brains. Br Med J, 289:1094, 1984

202. Potamianos G and Kellert JM: Anti-cholinergic drugs on memory; the effects of benzhexol on memory in a group of geriatric patients. Br J Psychiatry, 140:470-472, 1982

203. Goodwin JS and Regan M: Cognitive dysfunction associated with naproxen and ibuprofen the elderly. Arthritis Rheum, 25: 1013-1015, 1982

204. Garrison RH: Drug-nutrient interactions. In: 1984-85 Yearbook on Nutritional Medicine. Ed: J. Bland, Keats Publishing Inc, New Canaan, Connecticut, 1985

205. Carson R: Silent Spring. Houghton Miffin, Co., 1962

206. Tuormaa TE: Adverse effects of agrochemicals on reproduction and health: A brief review from the literature (Submission to the Pesticide Safety Directorate and Veterinary Medicines Directorate, March 1995). J Nutr & Environ Med, 5 (4): 353-366, UK, 1995

207. Nuttall N: Researchers blame DDT for world-wide fall in male fertility. The Times, 15th June, 1995

208. Cadbury D: The Feminization of Nature: Our future at risk. Penguin Books, 1997

209. Nuttall N: Scientists alarmed by sex-change of chemicals on men. The Times, 26th July, 1995

210. Brown P: Pesticides kill 40,000 a year says UN experts. The Guardian, 26th April, 1994

211. The London Food Commission: Food Adulteration and How to Beat It. Unwin Paperbacks, 1988

212. Nuttall N: Fruit and vegetables tainted with chemicals: Up to a quarter of lettuces may breach safety levels for fungicides. The Times, 3rd May, 1995

213. Nuttall N: Sheep dips linked to ill-health. The Times, 2nd July, 1999

214. Pesticides, Chemicals and Health: The BMA Guide Published on behalf of the British Medical Association by Edward Arnold, 1992

215. Purdey M: Are organophosphate pesticides involved in the causation of bovine spongiform encephalophaty (BSE)? Hypothesis based upon a literary review and limited trials on BSE cattle. J Nutr, Med, 4: 43-82, 1994

216. Evans M: Pesticides could have poisoned service personnel. The Times, 5th October, 1996

217. Evans: M: Gulf War pesticides linked to illness: Exposure to sprays could lead to brain damage. The Times, 17th November, 1997

218. Howard V: Synergistic effects of chemical mixtures – Can we rely on traditional toxicology? The Ecologist, 27 (5) 192-195, 1997

219. Abau-Donia MB et al: Neurotoxicity resulting from coexposure to pyridostigmine bromide, DEET and permethrin: Implications of Gulf War chemical exposure. J Toxicol and Environ Health, 48: 35-56, 1996

220. Brodie I: Gulf War troops 'poisoned'. The Times, 11th April, 1995

221. Latest BSE Update. Green Network News, February, 1997

222. Hornsby M: Ministry in U-turn on 'crank' farmer's mad cow theory. The Times, 13th April, 1998

223. By staff reporters: Britain exported suspected animal feeds. The Times, 13th June, 1996

224. Elliot V: BSE inquiry to cost £25m. The Times, 26th April, 1999

225. Hornsby M: Livestock fed most antibiotics. The Times, 7th December, 1998

226. Young R: Health risk as farms overuse antibiotics: Animals now harbour resistant organisms that could enter the food chain. The Times, 19th August,1999

227. Lees A and McVeigh K: An investigation of pesticide pollution in drinking water in England and Wales. Friends of the Eart Publications, 1988

228. Taylor G: Nitrates, nitrites, nitrosamines and cancer. Nutrition and Health, 2:47 1983

229. Sillanpaa M: FAO Soils Bulletin 63, Micronutrients assessment at the country level: An international study. FAO, Rome, 1990

230. Nuttall N: Health of the nation 'put at risk by factory farms'. The Times, 7th October, 1995

231. Hornsby M: Each family pays £1,000 to fund Euro farms. The Times, 1st July, 1994

232. Hornsby M: Ministers accused over food waste. The Times, 8th September, 1995

233. Sams C: Letters to the Editor, The Times, 7th September, 1997

234. A staff reporter: Organic diet linked to high sperm count. The Times, 10th June, 1994

235. Nuttall N and Elliott V: Doctors on alert from GM diseases. The Times, 25th May, 1999

236. Nuttall N: Bees 'spread genes from GM crops' – Ministers to review guidelines as new study shows that buffer zones may be futile. The Times, 15th May, 1999

237. Hawkes M and Nuttall N: Modified maize 'killing butterflies' – Catepillars are being poisoned by GM pollen. The Times, 10th May, 1999

238. Nuttall N: Silent spring 2020 – Genetically altered plants could wreak environmental havoc. The Times, 13th July, 1998

239. Gray G: Letters to the Editor. The Times, 28th May, 1999

240. Grove N: Air; an atmospheric of uncertainty. National Geographic, 17 (4): 503-536, 1997

241. Nuttall N: Promotion of green fuel failed to make a distinction between use with and without convererter – MPs seek inquiry into dangers of unleaded. The Times, 26th October, 1994

242. Nuttall N: Scientists predict increase in ozone – Exhaust cleaners will add smog problem in cities. The Times, 31st July, 1995

243. Nuttall N and Hawkes N: Diesel fumes 'are killing thousands of people a year'. The Times, 9th November, 1995

244. Dawe T: Millions face air of despair: A Times investigation into pollution and health of a nation. The Times, 10th January, 1994

245. Murray I: Heart attacks and traffic pollution linked in study. The Times, 5th August, 1997

246. Murray I: Air pollution 'hastens death of thousands'. The Times, 14th January, 1998

247. Laurance J: Deadly atmosphere claims lives in polluted cities. The Times, 9th December, 1993

248. Nuttall N: Price of traffic is put at £50bn. The Times, 4th April, 1996

249. Russel-Jones R: Letters to the Editor, The Times, 14th January, 1994

250. Prynn J: Public transport on obstacle course since privatisation. The Times, 30th January, 1997

251. Fresco A and Jenkins L: Mobile phone users 'face cancer risk', The Times, 3rd June, 1996

252. Nuttall N: Asthma rise is blamed on radio frequencies. The Times, 40th April, 1995

253. Murray I: VDU radiation making office workers sick: New evidence cuts symptoms ranging from runny nose to backache. The Times, 14th July, 1999

254. Nuttall N: Scientists trace cost of pollution to health. The Times, 20th July, 1995

255. Coleman V: Betrayal of Trust. European Medical Journal, PO Box 30, Barnstable, Devon EX32 9YU, 1994

256. Cousins N: Anatomy of Illness: as Perceived by the Patient. Bantam Books, London, New York, 1981

257. Gordon R: The Alarming History of Medicine. Sinclair-Stevenson, U.K., 1993

258. Illich I: Medical Nemesis: The Exropriation of Health. Calder & Boyers, UK. 1975

259. Medawar C: Power and Dependence: Social Audit on the Safety of Medicines. Social Audit Ltd, U.K., 1992

260. Thompson C and MacEoin D: The Health Crisis. The Natural Medicines Society, U.K.,1988

261. Hawkes N: Hospital drugs may be killing thousands a year. The Times, 15th April, 1998

262. Ashton H: Adverse effects of prolonged benzodiazepine use. Adverse Drugs Reaction Bulletin, No:118, June, 1986

263. Ashton H: Benzodiazepine withdrawal: an unfinished story. Br Med J, 288: 1135-1140, 1984

264. Breggin P: Toxic Psychiatry. Fontana Paperbags, London, 1993

265. Barton A: Taxpayers swallow a bitter pill. The Times, 19th April, 1994

266. Collier J: The Health Conspiracy. Century Hutchinson Ltd, 1989

267. Croce P: Vivisection or Science? – An investigation into testing drugs and safeguarding health. Zed Books Ltd, UK. 1999

268. The Pharmaceutical Drug Racket: Campaign Against Fraudulent Medical Research. PO Box 128, Carbramatta NSW 2166, Australia. 1993

269. Levine, R: Pharmocology: Drug Actions and Reactions. Little, Brown & Co. 1978

270. Kupsinel R: Vivisection: Science or Sham. PO Box 2102, Anaheim, California, 92814, US 1990

271. Richards G: Quantum Pharmacology. Butterworth, 1980

272. Ames BN, et al: Carcinogens and mutagens. A simple test system combining liver homogenates for activation and bacteria for detection. Proc Net Acad Sci, 70: 2281-5, 1973

273. Ruesh H: Slaughter of the Innocent: Animals in medical research. Futura Publications, UK. 1988

274. Murray I: Tamoxifen causes as well as cures cancer. The Times, 16th February, 1999

275. Hawkes N: Prescription for trouble when cures have a price. The Times, 5th October, 1995

276. Murray I: Britain trails Mexico in world health study. The Times, 3rd April, 1997

277. Laurance J: GPs wasting money on wrong drugs: Family doctors are over-prescribing to the tune of £425 million, with patients at risk, the Audit Commission has found. The Times, 8th March, 1994

278. Tuormaa TE: Psychoneuro-immunology. Soc for Environ Ther Newsletter, 10 (3&4): 138-142, 1990

279. Smith G: Placebo and belief system. Int J Alt & Compl Med, 17 (4): 9-10, 1999

280. McTaggart L: What Doctors don't Tell You: The truth about dangers of modern medicine. Thorsons, 1996

281. Chaitow L: Vaccination and Immunization: Dangers, Delusions and Alternatives (What every parent should know) CW Daniel Ltd, UK, 1999

282. Murray I: Measles vaccine's link with autism studied. The Times, 27th Febuary, 1998

283. Murray I: Researchers reject link between autism and trible vaccine: parent's groups are sceptical about government agency's reassurances. The Times, 11th June, 1999

284. Baraff L, et al: Possible temporal association between DPT vaccination and SIDS. Paed Inf Dis, 2 (1): 7, 1983

285. Coulter C and Fisher BL: "DPT: A shot in the Dark". Avery Publishing, New York, 1991

286. McTaggert L: What the medical profession fails to tell you. The Times, 19th August, 1997

287. Laurance J: Screening for breast cancer 'waste of money'. The Times, 30th June, 1995

288. Drife J: Is cervical screening really worthwhile? The Times, 17th October, 1995

289. Sweeney K: Fears and smears – When a cervical smear test reveals a minor abnormality, which is better: immmediate treatment, or constant surveillance? The Times, 21st October, 1994

290. Kennedy D: Hepatistis fear prompts call for patients to use own blood. The Times, 8th April, 1996

291. Murray I: Thousands infected in hospitals by lax hygiene standards. The Times, 15th May, 1997

292. Murray I: Hospital infections kill thousands: an instidius peril that now claims more lives that are lost on the roads. The Times, 16th September, 1997

293. Young R: Hospital food 'can make sick sicker'. The Times, 9th August, 1994

294. Strohman RC: Toward an epigenetic biology and medicine. Science and Medical Network Review, 57: 4-8, 1995

295. Wahlsten D: Intensitivity of the analysis of variance to heredity-environment interaction. Behav and Brain Sci, 13: 109-161, 1990

296. McKeown I: The Origin of Human Diseases. Basil Blackwell Inc., New York, 1988

297. Thoday JM: Letters to the Editor. The Times, 9th December, 1993

298. Payer Lynn: Medicine and Culture – Notions of Health and Sickness. Victor Gollancz, London, U.K., 1990

299. Cox IM, Cambell MJ and Dowson D: Red blood cell magnesium and chronic fatigue syndrome. The Lancet, 337: 757-760, 1991

300. Milton C: Doctors blame full wards on mentaly ill visitors. The Times, 22nd September, 1995

301. Hawkes N: Migraton linked to mental illness. The Times, 20th September, 1995

302. Letts Q: When ethnic origins cause mental health problems: on the official regonition of cultural ailments. The Times, 9th January, 1996

303. Murray I: Doctors accuse US of wrecking cancer drug test: researhers are angry that early announcement of results will ruin the trial. The Times, 8th April, 1998.

304. van Os J and Needleman J: Medicine in Europe: Caring for mentally ill people. Br Med J, 309: 1218-1221, 1994

305. Laurance J: Increased resistance to antibiotics raises risk of health crisis. The Times, 19th July, 1996

306. Cannon G: Superbug: Nature's Revenge. Virgin, U.K., 1995

307. Benjamin H: Everybody's Guide to Nature Cure. Health for All Publishing, Co, 1936

308. Barnes B and Bradley SG: Planning for a Healthy Baby: Essential Reading for all Future Parents. Ebury Press, 1990

309. Bradley SG and Bennett N: Preparation for Pregnancy: An Essential Guide. Argyll Publishing, 1995

310. Glenville M: Health Professionals' Guide to Preconception Care. Available from: Foresight, 28 The Paddock, Godalming, Surrey GU7 1XD.

311. Jennings IW: Vitamins and Endocrine Metabolism. William Heineman Medical Press, 1970

312. Bryce-Smith D: Pre-natal zinc deficiency. Nursing Times, pp 44-46, March, 1986

313. Stuttaford T: Zinc supplements improves babies' birth weight. The Times, 11th August, 1995

314. Steer P, et al: Relation between maternal haemoglobin concentration and birth weight in different ethnic groups. Br Med J: 310: 489-491, 1995

315. Odent M: A new page in the history of antenatal care. Primal Health Research, 2 (4): 3-7, 1995 Available from; 59 Roderick Road, London NW3 2NP, UK

316. Tuormaa TE: The adverse effects of manganese deficiency on reproduction and health: A literature review. J Orthomol Med, 11(2):69-79, 1996

317. Saner G, et al: Hair manganese concentrations in newborns and their mothers. Am J Clin Nutr, 41: 1042-1044, 1985

318. Kelsey JL et al: Maternal smoking and congenital malformations: An epidemiological study. Epidem Community Health, 32: 103-107, 1978

319. Rantakallio P, et al: Maternal smoking during pregnancy and delinquency of the offspring: an association without causation? Int J Epidemiol, 21: 1106-1113, 1992

320. Hemsworth BN: Deformation of the mouse foetus after ingestion of nicotine by the male. IRCS Medical Science, 9: 728-729, 1981

321. Hawkes N: Smoking fathers may sow seeds of cancer. The Times, 17th December, 1996

322. Parry M: How a father can harm his unborn child: New reserach warns men about drinking and smoking risks. Daily Express, 15th December, 1992

323. Tuormaa TE: Adverse effects of genito-urinary infections with particular reference to fertility and pre-conceptional care. J Nutr Med, 4 (3): 351-361, 1994

324. Laurance J: Infertility linked to rapid spread of infectious disease. The Times, 7th November, 1996

325. Ward NI, et al: Placental element levels in relation to fetal development for obstretically normal births: a study of 37 elements. Evidence for the effects of cadmium, lead and zinc on fetal growth and smoking as a cause of cadmium. Int J Biosocial Res, 9 (1): 63-81, 1987

326. Maugh TH: Hair: a diagnostic tool to complement blood serum and urine. Science, 202: 1271-1273, 1978

327. Laker M: On determining trace elements in man: to uses of blood and hair. Lancet, 31: 260-262, 1978

328. Bland J: Hair Tissue Mineral Analysis: An emergent diagnostic technique. Thorsons, UK, 1984

329. Tuormaa TE: Chromium, selenium and copper and other trace minerals in health and repoduction. J Orthomolecular Med, 15 (3): 145-156, 2000

330. Johnson HL and Sauberlich HE: Trace element analysis in biological samples. In: Clinical, Biochemical and Nutritional Aspects of Trace Elements (Ed AS Prasad) pp 405-426, Alan Liss Inc, New York, US 1982

331. Wolf WR: Trace element analysis in food. In: Clinical, Biochemical and Nutritional Aspects of Trace Elements (Ed AS Prasad) pp427-446, Alan Liss Inc, New York, US, 1982.

332. Borel JS, Anderson RA: Chromium. In: Biochemistry of the Essential Ultratrace Elements. (Ed E Frieden) Plenum Publishing Co, 1981

333. Ward N: Preconceptional care and pregnancy outcome. J Nutr & Environ Med, 5: 205-208, 1995

334. OPCS Congenital Malformation Satistics 1981-1985; Notifications, England and Wales. London Office of Population Censuses and Surveys Series MB3, No:2, London HMSO.

335. Hagberg B, et al: Decreasing perinatal mortality – increase in cerebral palsy morbidity? Acta Paediatrica Scandinavia, 78: 664-670, 1989

336. Pharoah POD, et al: Birthweight specific trends in cerebral palsy. Arch Dis Child, 65: 602-606, 1990

337. Rona RJ, et al: Effects of prematurity and intra-uterine growth on respiratory health and lung function in childhood. Br Med J, 306: 817-820, 1993

338. Crawford MA, et al: Nutrition and neurodevelopmental disorders. Nutrition and Health, 9: 81-97, 1993

339. Pharoah POD, et al: Prevalence of behaviour disorders in low birth weight infants. Arch Dis Child, 70: 271-274, 1994

340. Wortis H, et al: Deviant behaviour in 2 1/2 year-old children. Child Develop, 35: 871-879, 1964

341. Siegel LS: The long-term prognosis of pre-term infants. Conceptual, methodolical and ethical issues. Special Issue: Birth Management II, Human Nature, 5 (1): 103-126, 1994

342. Birch HG and Gussow JD: Disadvantaged Children: health nutrition and school failure. Harcour Brace, New York, US, 1970

343. Psychologic correlates of premature birth: A review J Nerv Ment Dis, 134: 129-144, 1962

344. Pasamanick B, et al: Pregnancy experience and the development of childhood speech disorders: An epiodemical study of the association with maternal and fetal factors. Am J Dis Child, 91: 113-118, 1956

345. Drillien CM: The Growth and Deveopment of Premature Infant. Williams & Wilkins, Baltimore, US, 1964

346. Barker DJP: Mothers, Babies and Disease in Later Life. BMJ Books, London, 1994

347. Barker DJP and Osmond C: Infant mortality, childhood nutrition and ischaemic heart disease in England and Wales. Lancet, i: 1977-1981, 1986

348. Barker DJP, et al: fetal nutrition and cardiovascuar disease in adult life. Lancet, 341:938-941, 1993

349. Osmond C, et al: Early growth and death from cardiovascular disease in women. Br Med J, 307: 1519-1524, 1993

350. Barker DJP, et al: Growth in utero and serum cholesterol concentrations in adult life. Br Med J, 307: 1524-1527, 1993

351. Benediktsson R, et al: Glucocorticoid exposure in utero: new model for adult hypertension. Lancet, 341: 339-341, 1993

352. Leon DA, et al: Failure to realise growth potential in utero and adult obesity in relation to blood pressure in 50 year old Swedish men. Br Med J, 312: 401-406, 1996

353. Hales CN, et al: Fetal infant growth and impaired glucose tolerance at age 64 years. Br Med J, 303: 1019-1022, 1991

354. Lithell HO, et al: Relation of size at birth to non-insulin dependent diabetes and insulin concentrations in men aged 50-60 years. Br Med J, 312: 406-410, 1996

355. Illman J: Britain's underfed babies the unhealthiest in Europe. The Observer, 19th April, 1998

356. Parliamentary Debates (Hansard), House of Lords Official Report, Vol:568, No: 23, HMSO, London, 1996

357. Murray I: World health crisis as West exports its lifestyle diseases. The Times, 5th May, 1997

358 Brown P: The dilemma that confronts the world: Water shortages, global warming and nitrogen pollution threaten planet's future unless politicians act now says UN environment expert. The Guardian, 16th Septemeber, 1999

359 Goldsmith E: Ultimate Freedom. Fourth World Review, 29: 6-11, 1999

360 Rothenberg D: Will the real Chief Seattle please speak up? In: The New Earth Reader, Ed: D Rothenberg and M Ulvaeus. The MIT Press, 1999

BIBLIOGRAPHY

Nutrition:

Melwyn R. Werbach, M.D.: Nutritional Influences on Illness: A sourcebook of clinical research. Thorsons, UK, 1988

Effective Nutritional Medicine: The Application of Nutrition to Major Health Problems. Published by British Society for Allergy Environmental and Nutritional Medicine (BSAENM), PO Box 7, Knighton LD7 1WT, UK, 1995

Jeffrey Bland (Ed): Yearbook of Nutritional Medicine 1984-85. Keats Publishing, New Canaan, CT, US, 1985

Dr Stephen Davies & Dr Alan Stewart A: Nutritional Medicine: The drug-free guide to better family health. Pan Books, UK, 1987

Sandra Goodman, PhD: Nutrition and Cancer: Sate of the Art. Green Library, UK, 1995

Dr David Horrobin (Ed): Clinical Uses of Essential Fatty Acids. Eden Press, Montreal, Canada, 1982

Matti Tolonen: Vitamins and Minerals in Health and Nutrition. Ellis Horwood Ltd, 1990

Dr Abram Hoffer: A Guide to Eating well for Pure Health. Quarry Press, PO Box 1061, Ontario K7L 4Y5, Canada

Dr Linus Pauling: How to Live Longer and Feel Better. W.H. Freeman, N.Y. US, 1986

Patrick Holford: The Optimum Nutrition Bible. Piatkus, UK, 1998

Professor John Yudkin: Pure, White and Deadly – A Problem of Sugar. Viking, London, UK, 1987

Martin Budd: Low Blood Sugar – The 20th Century Epidemic. Thorsons, UK, 1983

Paavo Airola: Hypoglycaemia: A Better Approach. Health Plus Publishers, Phoenix, Arizona, US, 1977

Nutritional Psychiatry:

Merwyn R. Werbach, M.D.: Nutritional Influences on Mental Illness: A sourcebook of clinical research. Third Line Press, Tarzana, CA, US, 1991

Phospholipid Spectrum Disorder in Psychiatry. Eds: M. Peet, I. Glen and D. Horrobin. Marius Press Carnfort, 1999

Carl C. Pfeiffer, PhD, M.D: Mental and Elemental Nutrients: A Physician's guide to Nutrition and Health Care. Keaths Publishing, New Canaan, CT, US, 1975

Biological Aspects of Schizophrenia and Addiction. Ed: Gwynneth Hemmings. John Wiley & Sons, 1982

William H Philpott & Dwight K Kalita: Brain Allergies: The psycho-nutrient connection. Keats Publishing, New Canaan, CT, US, 1980

Dr Michael Lesser: Nutrition & Vitamin Therapy: The Dietary Treatment for Mental and Emotional Ill-health. Thorsons, UK, 1980

Dr Abram Hoffer & Dr Morton Walker: Smart Nutrients: A Guide to Nutrients That can Reverse Senility. Avery Publishing, N.Y., US, 1994

Tuula E Tuormaa: An Alternative to Psychiatry. The Book Guild Ltd, UK, 1991

Patrick Holford & Carl C. Pfeiffer, PhD, M.D: Mental Health: The Nutrition Connection – Mental Illness: The Nutrition Connection. ION Press, UK, 1996

Food/chemical Allergy:

Professor Jonathan Brostoff & Linda Gamlin: The Complete Guide to Food Allergy and Intolerance. Bloomsbury, UK, 1998

Effective Allergy Practice: A document on standard care and management for the allergy patient. Published by The British Society for Allergy Environmental and Nutritional Medicine (BSAENM), PO Box 7, Knighton LD7 1WT, UK, 1994

Theron G. Randolph, M.D. & Ralph W. Moss, PhD: Allergies, Your Hidden Enemy: How the new field of Clinical Ecology can unravel the environmental causes of mental and physical illness. Thorsons, UK, 1981

Dr Richard Mackarness: Not All in the Mind. Pan Books, UK, 1990

Dr Keith Mumby: Allergy Handbook: A Doctor's Guide to Successful Treatment. Thorsons, UK, 1988

Dr John Mansfield: Arthritis – Allergy, Nutrition and Environment. Thorsons, UK 1995

William J. Rea, M.D.: Chemical Sensitivity, Vol.1,
Boca Raton, CRC Press, Chemical Sensitivity, Vol.2-4, Lewis Publishers, US, 1992

Childhood Hyperactivity:

Belinda Barnes & Vicky Colquhoun: The Hyperactive Child: Attention Deficit Hyperactivity Disorder: A practical self- help guide for parents. Thorsons, UK, 1997

Doris J. Rapp, M.D.: Is This Your Child? William Morrow, N.Y, US, 1991

Juvenile Delinquency:

Barbara Reed, PhD.: Food, Teens and Behaviour. Natural Press, PO Box 2107, Manitowoc, US, 1983

Alexander Schauss: Diet, Crime and Delinquency. Parker House, Berkeley, CA, US, 1981

Preconception Care:

Belinda Barnes & Suzanne Gail Bradley: Planning for a Healthy Baby: Essential Reading for all Future Parents. Ebury Press, UK, 1990

Suzanne Gail Bradley & Nicholas Bennett: Preparation for Pregnancy: An Essential Guide. Argyll Publishing, UK, 1995

Margaret Wynn & Arthur Wynn: The Case for Preconception of Men and Women. AB Academic Publishers, Bicester, Oxford, UK, 1991

Marilyn Glenville: Natural Solutions to Infertility. Piatkus, UK, 2000

General Interest:

Pietro Croce: Vivisection or Science? An investigation into testing drugs and safeguarding health. Zed Books Ltd, London, UK, 1999

Hans Ruesch: Slaughter of the Innocent: Animals in medical research. CIVITAS Publications, 1991.

Gordon Moran: Silencing Scientists and Scholars in Other Fields: Power, padagrim controls, peer review and scholarly communication. Ablex, US, 1998

Dr Joe Collier: The Health Conspiracy: How doctors, the drug industry and the government undermine our health. Century Hutchinson, UK, 1989

Lynne McTaggart: What Doctors Don't Tell You: The truth about the dangers of modern medicine. Thorsons, UK, 1996

Leon Chaitow: Vaccination and Immunization: Dangers, Delusions and Alternatives (What Every Parent Should Know) C.W Daniel Ltd, UK, 1999

Charles Medawar: Power and Dependence – Social Audit on the safety of medicines. Social Audit Ltd, PO Box 111, London NW1 8XG, UK, 1992

Dr Vernon Coleman: Betrayal of Trust. Publishing House, Trinity Place, Barnstable, Devon EX32 9HJ, UK, 1994

Lynne Payer: Medicine and Culture: Notions of Health and Sickness. Victor Gollancz Ltd, UK, 1989

Geoffrey Cannon: Superbug: Nature's Revenge. Virgin, UK, 1995

Caroline Walker & Geoffrey Cannon: The Food Scandal. Century Publishing, UK, 1985

The BMA Guide to Pesticides, Chemicals and Health. Edward Arnold, 1992

Deborah Cadbury: The Feminization of Nature: Our Future at Risk. Penguin Books, 1998

Dr Cyril Smith and Simon Best: Electromagnetic Man – Health and hazard in the electrical environment. St Martin's Press, NY, US, 1988

John Robbins: Reclaiming your Health: Exploding the medical myth and embracing the source of true healing. HJ Kramer Inc, US, 1998

Michael Crawford & David March: The Driving Force: Food in Evolution and Future. Mandarin, UK, 1991

Edward Goldsmith: The Way: An ecological world-view. Themis Books, London, UK, 1996

Journals:

Journal of Nutritional & Environmental Medicine. Carfax Publishing Company, PO Box 25, Abingdon, Oxfordshire OX14 3UE, UK.

Journal of Orthomolecular Medicine. 16 Florence Avenue, Toronto, Ontario, Canada M2N 1E9

Nutrition and Health. AB Academic Publishers, POB 42, Bicester, Oxon OX6 7NW, UK.

The Nutrition Practitioner. 51 Trevelyan, Bracknell RG12 8YD, UK.

The Ecologist. Unit 18, Chelsea Wharf, Lots Road, London SW10 0QJ, UK.

What Doctors Don't Tell You. 77 Grosvenor Avenue, London N5 2NN, UK.

Environment & Health News. 86-88 Colston Street, Bristol BS1 5BB, UK.

Pesticides News (The Journal of The Pesticides Trust) Eurolink Centre, 49 Effra Road, London SW2 IBZ, UK.

Electromagnetic Hazard & Therapy. PO Box 2039, Shoreham by Sea, BN43 5JD, UK.

The Food Magazine: Campaign for safer, healtier food. The Food Commission, 94 White Lion Street, London N1 9PF, UK.

Health Consciousness Magazine P.O. Box 550, Oviedo, FL 32765, US.

Total Health in Today's World. PO Box 60042, Potomac, Maryland 20859-0042, US.

HEAL. PO Box 29629, Atlanta, GA 30359, US.

WorldWatch, 1776 Massachusetts Ave, NW, Washington, DC 20036, US.

Nexus Magazine. PO Box 30, Mapleton, Qld 4560, Australia

Useful Addresses: (Please enclose SAE)

Foresight – The Association for the Promotion of Preconceptual Care. 28 The Paddock, Godalming, Surrey GU7 1XD.

HACSG – The Hyperactive Children's Support Group. 71 Wyke Lane, Chichester, West Sussex PO19 2LD.

British Association of Nutritional Therapists (BANT), London WC1N 3XX Tel: 0870 6061284

British Society for Allergy Environmental and Nutritional Medicine (BSAENM), PO Box 7, Knighton LD7 1WT.

General Council and Register of Naturopaths. Goswell House, 2 Goswell Road, Street, Somerset BA16 0JG.

The Schizophrenia Association of Great Britain (SAGB). Bryn Hyfryd, The Cresent, Bangor, Gwynedd LL57 2AG.

The Institute of Optimum Nutrition (I.O.N.) Blades Court, Deodar Road, London SW15 2NU, Tel: 020 8877 9993

The Hale Clinic & The Nutri Centre. 7 Park Creset, London W1N 3HE, Tel: 020 7436 5122 (For supplement orders & advice) 020 7323 2382 (The bookshop)

AAA – Action Against Allergy. PO Box 278, Twickenham, Middlesex TW1 4QQ.

The McGarrison Society: The Institute of Brain Health and Human Nutrition, Hackney Hospital, Homerton High Street, London E9 6BE, UK.

The Environmental Medicine Foundation. c/o Pamela Ross, Rickmansworth, Herts WD3 5SP

The Scientific and Medical Network. Gibliston Mill, Colinsburgh, Leven, Fife, Scotland KY9 1JS

Green Network. 9 Clairmont Road, Lexden, Colchester CO3 5BE, UK.

Women's Environmental Network. Unit 30, Aberdeen Studios, 22 Highbury Grove, London N5 2EA, Tel: 020 7704 6800

The Food Commission (Consumer watchdog on food). 94 White Lion Street, London N1 9PF. Tel:020 7837 2250,

The Soil Association. Bristol House, 40-56 Victoria Street, Bristol BS1 6BY (Organic food regulatory body which can supply names and addresses of organic retail outfits in Britain) Tel: 0117 929 0661, Fax: 0117 925 2504

Organics Direct. 1-7 Willow Street, London WC2A 4BH. National delivery of organic produce. Call for free brochure: 020 7729 2828

Pure Organics Ltd, Stockport Farm, Amesbury, Wilts. SP4 7LN Tel: 01980 626263

SimplyOrganic Food Company. A62-A64 New Covent Garden Market. London SW8 5YY. Call for free brocure: 0870 162 3010

Compassion in World Farming (CIWF), Charles House, 5A Charles Street, Petersfield, Hampshire GU32 3EH

GeneWatch UK, The Courtyard, Whitecross Road, Tideswell, Buxton, Derbyshire SK17 8NY. Tel: 01298 871898 Fax: 01298 872531

Action Against Pesticide Exposure (PEGS). Eurolink Centre, 49 Effra Road, London SW2 1BZ

Additives Survival Network (UK). 63 Downland Road, Devizes, Wilts. SN10 5EF.

JABS (vaccination/immunisation). 1 Gawsworth Road, Golbourne, Warrington WA3 3RF.

The Informed Parent. PO Box 870, Harrow, Middx HA3 7UW.

NEMESIS Light on Medical Fraud. 1 Quarry Bank Road, Chesterfield S41 0HH.

British Antivivisection Association (BAVA). PO Box 73, Chesterfield S41 0YZ

U.K. Anti-vivisection Information Service (UKAVIS). PO Box 4746, London SE11 4XF

People for the Ethical Treatment of Animals (PETA). Lindburn House, 324 Kilburn High Road, London NW6 2QJ

Dr Hadwen Trust – Medical Research without Animal Experiemnts, Dr Hadwen House, 84A Tilehouse Street, Hitchin, Herts SG5 2DY. Tel: 01462 436819 Fax: 01462 4368444

Doctors and Lawyers for Resposible Medicine (DLRM). 104b Weston Park, London N8 9PP. Tel: 020 8340 9813, Fax: 020 8342 9878

National Pure Water Association. 12 Dennington Lane, Crigglestone, Wakefield WF4 3ET.

Transport 2000. Walkden House, 10 Melton Street, London NW1 2EJ.

Friends of the Earth. 26-28 Underwood Street, London N1 7JQ. Tel: 020 7490 1555

Greenpeace. Canonbury Villas, London N1 2PN. Tel: 020 7865 8100

INDEX

191